Intermittent Fasting Mastery

2 Manuscripts:
Intermittent Fasting for Women,
Intermittent Fasting 16/8

Jenna Dawson

Intermittent Fasting Mastery

Written by Jenna Dawson

First Edition

Copyrights Notice

Limited Liability

Please note that the content of this book is based on personal experience and various information sources.

Although the author has made every effort to present accurate, up-to-date, reliable, and complete information in this book, they make no representations or warranties concerning the accuracy or completeness of the content of this book and specifically disclaim any implied warranties of merchantability or fitness for a particular purpose.

Your particular circumstances may not be suited to the example illustrated in this book; in fact, they likely will not be. You should use the information in this book at your own risk.

All trademarks, service marks, product names, and the characteristics of any names mentioned in this book are considered the property of their respective owners and are used only for reference. No endorsement is implied when we use one of these terms.

This book is only for personal use. Please note the information contained within this document is for educational and entertainment purposes only and no warranties of any kind are declared or implied. Readers acknowledge that the author is not engaged in providing medical, dietary, nutritional, or professional advice, or physical training.

Please consult a doctor, nutritionist or dietician, before attempting any techniques outlined in this book. Nothing in this book is intended to replace common sense or medical consultation or professional advice and is meant only to inform.

By reading this book, the reader agrees that under no circumstances is the author responsible for any losses, direct or indirect, which are incurred as a result of the use of the information contained within this document, including, but not limited to, errors, omissions, or inaccuracies.

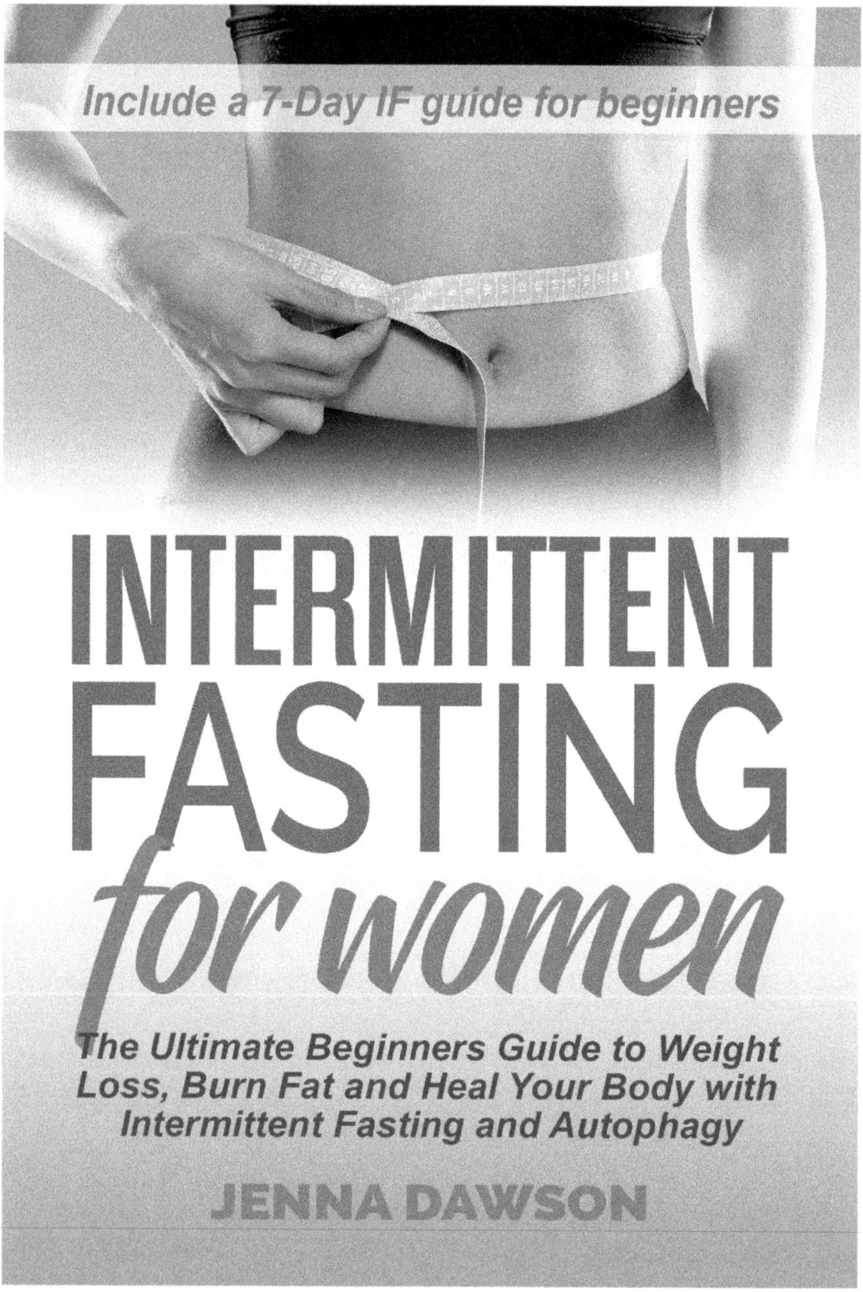
Include a 7-Day IF guide for beginners
INTERMITTENT
FASTING
for women
The Ultimate Beginners Guide to Weight Loss, Burn Fat and Heal Your Body with Intermittent Fasting and Autophagy
JENNA DAWSON

page intentionally left blank

Intermittent Fasting for Women

The Ultimate Beginners Guide to Weight Loss, Burn Fat and Heal Your Body with Intermittent Fasting and Autophagy

Jenna Dawson

Intermittent Fasting for Women

Written by Jenna Dawson

First Edition

Copyrights Notice

Limited Liability

Please note that the content of this book is based on personal experience and various information sources.

Although the author has made every effort to present accurate, up-to-date, reliable, and complete information in this book, they make no representations or warranties concerning the accuracy or completeness of the content of this book and specifically disclaim any implied warranties of merchantability or fitness for a particular purpose.

Your particular circumstances may not be suited to the example illustrated in this book; in fact, they likely will not be. You should use the information in this book at your own risk.

All trademarks, service marks, product names, and the characteristics of any names mentioned in this book are considered the property of their respective owners and are used only for reference. No endorsement is implied when we use one of these terms.

This book is only for personal use. Please note the information contained within this document is for educational and entertainment purposes only and no warranties of any kind are declared or implied. Readers acknowledge that the author is not engaged in providing medical, dietary, nutritional, or professional advice, or physical training.

Please consult a doctor, nutritionist or dietician, before attempting any techniques outlined in this book. Nothing in this book is intended to replace common sense or medical consultation or professional advice and is meant only to inform.

By reading this book, the reader agrees that under no circumstances is the author responsible for any losses, direct or indirect, which are incurred as a result of the use of the information contained within this document, including, but not limited to, errors, omissions, or inaccuracies.

Table of Contents

Introduction 18

Chapter 1 20

- What is Intermittent Fasting (IF)? 21
- History of Intermittent Fasting 22
- How does Intermittent Fasting work? 23
- Two IF states: Fed Vs. Fasted 24
- Fat-Adaptation 25
- How is Intermittent Fasting different from dieting? 27

Chapter 2 30

- Why change your eating patterns? 31
- Does IF affect behavior? 32
- Health benefits of Intermittent Fasting 34
- Therapeutic benefits of Intermittent Fasting 38
- 3 Famous Intermittent Fasting schedules 39
- Daily Intermittent Fasting 40
- Weekly Intermittent Fasting 42
- Alternate Day Intermittent Fasting 43
- Strategies of IF that proved most beneficial for women 45
- How to get started with Intermittent Fasting? 53

Chapter 3 56

- Design your own IF program 57
- Protocols necessary to succeed in Intermittent Fasting 59
- Significance of fluids during Intermittent Fasting 63

Helpful tips for Intermittent Fasting 65
How to use Intermittent Fasting for muscle gain? 71
Common mistakes to avoid during Intermittent Fasting 73
Precautionary measures for Intermittent Fasting 80
Female hormonal balance and Intermittent Fasting 83
How does IF affect women differently than men? 85
Chapter 4 88
When should women avoid Intermittent Fasting? 89
Pros and cons of IF for women 90
7-Day Intermittent Fasting Guide for Beginners 90
Is Exercise Safe for women during IF? 102
Chapter 5 106
Why is Autophagy important for women? 107
Keys to improving general health 110
How does Intermittent Fasting prevent cancer? 117
IF makes healthy eating simpler and easier 118
Chapter 6 120
Tips to ease through intermittent fast 121
Research-proven advantages of IF for women 123
Reviews from women who practiced Intermittent Fasting 127
Women who tried Intermittent Fasting for a week 127
The woman who tried Intermittent Fasting for 8 months 128
Conclusion 130
Final words on Intermittent Fasting for women 131

Introduction

The world itself bears witness to the fact that many fitness and health trends have come and gone. Some catch the attention of the people and stay in trend for long periods like yoga while some of them draw immediate attention but lose the charm over time because of difficulty levels or side-effects.

Everyone wants to be healthy, fit and wants to look attractive. And to do this, some people adopt the way of exercising and workouts while some people follow strict diet plans. In both scenarios, the purpose is to achieve goal weight, increase physical health, and develop a peaceful state of mind.

Diets are pretty common in this day and age. They are more popular than any other weight-loss techniques.

Men and women of all ages indulge in dieting but a majority of them ends up with nutritional deficiencies and with worse health condition than before. Diets limit the calorie intake of the day and this makes it difficult for you to meet the nutritional needs of the body. And this is where fasting comes in!

Fasting is the most popular and widely known technique known to humans for hundreds of centuries now. In some parts of the world, it is followed as a religious obligation like Christianity and Islam; while in others it is used as a natural and easy weight-loss tool.

It can be used as both and humans all over the world can profit from this natural technique; no matter from which culture or race they belong to.

One of the most popular, easy, and healthy fitness trends is 'Intermittent Fasting'. By following this technique, you will not only lose weight and burn the fats but you will also nourish and heal your body. In other words, it is the healthiest way of losing weight known to man yet. It is also the easiest technique since it doesn't require extremely tough gym workouts or mind tormenting hunger levels. Anyone can apply this technique to their lives because it doesn't need special efforts or time.

It is most beneficial for women because they do not have any extra time while juggling work and home duties. Intermittent Fasting is proven the most effective and most commonly adopted fitness technique by women all over the world.

Chapter 1

What is Intermittent Fasting (IF)?

The word 'Intermittent' has a literal meaning of 'an occurrence at non-continuously and irregular intervals'. Fasting means to 'abstain from a certain activity for a defined period'.

'Intermittent Fasting' simply implies refraining from eating food for a certain defined time. There are two aspects of Intermittent Fasting:

- **Fasting window** – Period in which you abstain from eating.
- **Feeding window** – Period in which you are allowed to eat.

The fasting window is defined by you and you decide which hours of the day or which days of the week you can easily fast. If you are comfortable with a daily fast then you define major hours of the day as your 'fasting window'.

During your fasting window, you are not allowed to eat anything. Anyway, there's no limit on fluid intake though. You can drink fluids as much you want during your fast. The best and suitable drinks for fasting will be discussed later.

The feeding window is known as those hours of the day when you are not under a fast and you can eat anything you want in this window. Unlike diets, there is no restriction on what to eat.

As long as you eat healthy and fresh, you can have just about anything. During the feeding window, you meet the nutritional needs of your body and make up for the nutrition and energy that you took from it.

'Feeding window' has a range between 8 to 12 hours depending upon your stamina. Usually, it's a good practice to start with a long feeding window and a shorter fasting window and then you gradually increase your fasting window and decrease the feeding window.

Intermittent Fasting (IF) is an eating pattern where your body cycles between periods of fasting and eating: so, this concept is based on voluntary abstinence from food for certain periods. Humans are designed and are well able to perform intermittent fasts.

Intermittent Fasting is a technique that anyone can implement as well as alter or change according to his/her routine. It focuses on stabilizing the times of eating which helps the body to get maximum energy out of a meal.

It is not the only weight-loss program out there but it is the healthiest one. Other weight-loss programs can include extreme starvation and deprivation from healthy fats, but Intermittent Fasting is the only weight-loss technique that focuses on providing nourishment and health to your body.

History of Intermittent Fasting

Humans have been fasting for thousands of years. Sometimes they did it due to religious obligations and sometimes just because there wasn't enough food. In the early history of humankind, when there was a shortage of food, people used to perform extended fasts.

They did not have access to an abundance of food and had food barely enough to survive. That is why; 'Intermittent Fasting' holds the title of the most ancient food practice in human history.

Now, although we live in a world where we see an abundance of food, still a large population deliberately avoids eating food for longer periods and the intent is to lose weight.

Researchers have conducted numerous studies and surveys and have found that tons of thousands of people from all around the world practice Intermittent Fasting weekly.

Some religions put an obligation on their followers too fast while the majority of people are in a race to lose fat mass, shedding extra pounds, and thus improve their body composition.

Indeed, Intermittent Fasting is now gaining popularity in weight-loss and bodybuilding communities, but it is not a new technique. It has been used by humans since the 1900s and it therapeutically treated many diseases like epilepsy, diabetes, and also obesity.

In modern-day time, Intermittent Fasting is attracting the attention of scientists as well as celebrities alike.

While scientists are conducting extensive researches on its benefits and using it as a medical aid in the health field, celebrities are looking for effective and best ways to attain a perfect and inspiring shape of the body.

How does Intermittent Fasting work?

Our body can handle extended periods of not eating. Human bodies have the natural ability to transition between the hunger state and the full state. When we don't eat for a long period, the processes going inside our body change.

When we eat our body starts to work on digesting it and storing the energy received through the meal. When we are hungry, our body starts to take energy from those stored fats.

When we fast for a specific time, our blood sugar and insulin levels face a reduction in their levels. It is normal because it pushes our bodies to thrive from existing resources present inside our bodies.

Researches have shown that fasting helps to protect against diseases like heart diseases, diabetes, cancer, and Alzheimer's disease.

Therefore, when in a fasted state, you shouldn't worry that it will affect your health.

To understand how Intermittent Fasting works, two states have to be understood first. The two states are – the fed state and the fasted state. By understanding these states, we get to know how our bodies keep functioning well although our stomachs are empty or full.

Two IF states: Fed Vs. Fasted

In the **Fed state**, the body is undergoing the process of digesting and absorbing food.

The state begins when you start eating and can last from three to five hours after that. In a fed state, your body shows elevated levels of insulin, and this acts as a signal for your body to store the excess amounts of calories.

This storage takes place in the fat cells. During the time with high insulin levels, the process of fat burning comes to a stop, and the body shifts towards burning glucose from your last meal instead.

Then a state called *post-absorptive* state comes, which lasts about 8 to 12 hours after the last meal. After that, the body enters the **Fasted state**. In the *Fasted state*; the body is not processing any meal and the levels of insulin are low.

This induces a mobilization of stored body fat presiding inside the body in the fat cells and starts to burn these fats for providing energy to the body. In this state, the body can burn the fat that was first inaccessible to it during the fed state.

Staying hungry for a specific duration of time helps you with hundreds of things. When you eat a meal, your body is under 'fed state' and is just processing the meal you just ate.

After a few hours pass and the food is completely digested, it goes into a mid-stage where you don't feel hungry but you haven't eaten anything else yet. You can call this an intermediate state.

After 8 to 12 hours from your last meal, a state comes called 'fasted state' when you feel hungry and you are under a fast. In this state, your body needs to re-gain the fuel to work but it doesn't find any energy being provided to it.

So, it starts to look for energy sources inside the body. It starts to go towards the fat cells where fats from your previous meals have been stored.

The body is designed to store some amount of fat from every meal to regain energy at the time when it is needed.

Thus, because of low insulin levels now the body has entered into a fat-burning state and it starts to burn the fats present inside the body.

This is beneficial in hundreds of ways. It will not only get rid of the excess fat from you but will also get rid of any toxins present inside a body.

The toxins can be anything harmful present in your body. It can be a dysfunctional cell or a cell that is damaged and is not performing well. Removal of such cells is very necessary when we talk about maintaining health.

So, you have to be under the 'fasted state' so that your body can initialize the burn-off state. Intermittent Fasting provides you a convenient way to enter into the fasted state and get rid of all excess fats, calories, and damaged cells.

Many health practitioners and doctors advise their patients to start fasting for this purpose. They believe that health will improve if they fast because of this quality of Intermittent Fasting.

Fat-Adaptation

Nature has given humans the ability to fuel their bodies with stored body-fat instead of glucose and extra calories. Just a little time and practice are needed to achieve the goal of regulating your metabolism based on existing resources in your body and let your body adapt to fat-burning pathways.

This practice is called *Fat-adaptation*. It includes improving your body's sensitivity to lower insulin levels and promoting mobilization of the fat from fat cells so that the body leans towards extracting energy from fat reserves inside the body instead of depending on constant fat resources being given to it externally through food.

At first, a person might perceive that this fasting technique is hard since it requires you to stay away from food in some portions of the day. But it is a wrong perception.

Intermittent Fasting does not stop or change what you eat; it just changes when you eat it. It has already been proven that eating too much or having large meals slows your metabolism, increases laziness, and reduces the productivity of a person.

Eating small portions of food at appropriate times of the day not only gives you higher energy levels but also boosts your metabolism and thus your body keeps getting healthier.

Thus, to burn the existing fat in your body, the fasted state has to be achieved. Your body will itself take energy from calories and fats already presiding in your body and that's how the fat is naturally burned away from our bodies.

Fasting puts the body in a state of burning fat and we cannot enter the fasted state until 8 to 12 hours from the last meal. This time is different for everyone since it depends on the metabolism rate.

It is important to practice the learning curve and you will get your body on track naturally.

How is Intermittent Fasting different from dieting?

Intermittent Fasting is not a diet in the conventional sense; in fact, it is a pattern of eating. It is a technique where you schedule your meals so that you and your body can get the most out of them.

Unlike diet plans, Intermittent Fasting does not focus on what to eat and what not to eat. This phenomenon emphasizes when to eat so that it may prove beneficial to your body.

Despite what some people may think, Intermittent Fasting is a fairly easy technique. Studies have been conducted in this regard and the majority of people have reported that they have higher energy levels during the fasting periods of the day.

The biggest difference between dieting and fasting is that dieting makes you stick to specific foods only and Intermittent Fasting keeps the options open for your stomach. You can enjoy whole meals filled with nutrition, protein, and even some healthy fats.

Diets like low-carb diets make you eat empty carbs and this does not provide any nutrition to your body. Human bodies specifically the female body needs all possible nutrition to stay healthy and fit.

And if you restrict your food intake to only a few foods, you will never be able to achieve a healthy and sound body.

Another difference between the two is Effectiveness in the same period. Dieting has proved very beneficial for some individuals and they claim they lost about 10 or 15lbs in one week.

But this comes at a heavy cost - losing sleep, facing anger problems due to starvation, and an overall bitterness to the personality and nature.

This happens because you are not naturally allowing the body to reduce fat; in fact, you are forcing your body to go through states which it generally won't go through.

On the other hand, Intermittent Fasting takes a much natural and consistent approach towards weight loss. It might take more time than conventional dieting, but it won't take a negative toll on your mind or health.

It won't induce anger or anxiety due to extreme hunger levels; instead, it will take a rather slower approach to get rid of the access fat from your body naturally.

One major difference between the two is Consistency. You can never follow diet plans for more than a few months or even a year.

After that, you get annoyed and go right back to your old eating habits and gain the lost weight back in no time.

This is something that pushes people into severe depression and they end up gaining more weight than they originally had.

Intermittent Fasting offers an easy to follow and convenient method to achieve your goal weight. You can make a permanent lifestyle out of it, adapt it as long as you want and you never have to give it up because of difficulty.

It is a very simple technique, does not require much effort or time.

Flexibility is another difference between the two. Dieting specifically tells you what foods to eat and avoid what foods.

Everyone has to follow the same instructions, eat specific foods, tediously counting, and limiting calorie intake. It is not at all flexible, meaning you cannot enjoy a pizza or a piece of cake every once in a while, because you will gain back the lost pounds.

IF on the other hand is flexible and every individual can tailor and customize it according to himself.

You can set eating times according to your will and ease, you don't have to face extreme restrictions on what foods to eat.

You are allowed to eat just about everything; you just have to follow a healthy schedule of when to eat.

Chapter 2

Why change your eating patterns?

The reason why Intermittent Fasting is so widely popular is that it doesn't require abstaining from food; it just demands healthier eating time patterns. Isn't it better to just eat at specific times instead of putting yourself through the miseries of extreme dieting rules? Instead of worrying about fats in different foods and counting calories before eating and being unable to relish your favorite foods, just adjust the patterns of eating and still enjoy a healthy body weight. Just tweak your schedule of eating and the job is done. That simple!

Intermittent Fasting is the simplest strategy to lose weight. It doesn't put a stress toll on your mind and stomach because of staying hungry. It also doesn't demand a drastic change in lifestyle or behavior. It is simple enough for anyone to implement it; yet so meaningful that it will make a difference.

This phenomenon simply takes excess weight from your body while keeping on the good weight on which helps you feel energetic throughout your day.

Diets are easy to contemplate but difficult to execute. The fast results of a diet appeal to everyone, but when you get into it, it becomes very tough very early. Suppose, you decide that you are going on a low-carb diet, a major portion of delicious and appealing foods have to be avoided.

Also, after staying hungry for long durations, you have to force yourself to eat foods that you don't want to eat all the time.

Whereas in Intermittent Fasting, you are not restricted on choices of food, you are just challenged to maintain proper eating times and patterns.

Thus, to conclude, the diet requires work than fasting. In a diet, you not only stay hungry but also you don't get to eat what you like. But in Intermittent Fasting, you just have to follow a schedule of eating and never have to worry about what to eat and what not to eat. Therefore, ease of Intermittent Fasting is intriguing to lose weight. Because it is easy to contemplate as well as execute.

It also provides a huge range of health benefits that a diet can never provide. Unlike a diet, IF doesn't snatch away nutrition from your body, that's why it keeps you healthy.

Moreover, a diet requires a massive change in lifestyle and eating habits. Intermittent Fasting is easy to implement and never demands huge alterations and modifications in lifestyle.

Does IF affect behavior?

Behaviors classify into two categories- health behaviors and personality behaviors. Let's see how does Intermittent Fasting affects both behaviors and does it enhance the quality of life or not?

Health behaviors*:* Intermittent Fasting has proved to help improve and modify different health behaviors like calorie intake, energy expenditure, and sleep. Calorie intake means how much you eat and energy expenditure refers to how much you move.

A balance between both of them is necessary to provoke a healthy lifestyle and an active body. If you eat too much and move less, it will only affect your health negatively and might act as the biggest drawback to your extra weight. The reverse of this case is also true.

If you exert a lot of energy during the day but then have an extremely heavy and large meal, this will also slow your metabolism rate and as a result, you will gain weight.

The last meal before sleeping must be a small meal so that your body can digest it before you sleep and this will allow your body to enter a state of fasting. This nightly fasting will decrease your calorie intake and will produce a significant decrease in weight. In return, this improves: Energy levels and sleep satisfaction.

Intermittent Fasting also reduces untimely snacks during the night and decreases the nighttime intake of food which enhances the quality of sleep.

Poor sleep quality leads to the risk of obesity, diabetes, and many heart-related diseases. Therefore, Intermittent Fasting plays a significant role in improving health behaviors thus giving you a healthier lifestyle.

Personality Behaviors: When you suddenly put your body through huge gaps in food intake during dieting and do not provide necessary nutrients like protein and healthy carbs, your body enters a state of constant exhaustion and fatigue.

This induces a state of stress on your body and indirectly it's you who face the stress and exhaustion.

The will to work is reduced, your energy levels drop and you find yourself in the mood to lie down and do minimize your activities.

Not moving enough and lying around makes your body habitual of the constant rest state and makes you lazy.

You don't want to walk, talk, work, or participate in social activities. You start becoming an introvert and that's how your whole personality shifts due to the drastic change in your diet.

Intermittent Fasting presents the best solution for this.

Intermittent Fasting does not induce massive and drastic changes in your diet plans. It slowly and steadily brings your body towards a schedule to eat at healthy times.

This allows your body to extract maximum energy out of it and you feel energized for longer durations of time.

You stay healthy, happy, and active. You start to work more, stay more active thus your physical, as well as mental health, improves. This fasting technique which defines windows of eating, not only improves your mental health which accounts for personality behaviors.

It also puts your body on a healthier path, and over time, you learn the best eating patterns that suit your lifestyle and personality.

Intermittent Fasting works for every person because it allows the ease of implementation.

If your job requires you to work all night and you sleep in the day, Intermittent Fasting offers a relaxed schedule to maintain suiting your requirements. You can define your window of eating and adjust accordingly.

Health benefits of Intermittent Fasting

Numerous studies conducted link Intermittent Fasting to substantial benefits for one's body, as well as the brain.

The following list includes some of the most important evidence-backed advantages of Intermittent Fasting:

1) Weight loss and burning belly fat: A major cause behind people, and especially women, taking up Intermittent Fasting is their concern for and the desire to lose weight and burn as much belly fat as possible. Since Intermittent Fasting requires one to eat fewer meals, it automatically reduces the calorie intake.

Furthermore, it enhances the body's metabolic rate by 3.6 – 14% by lowering insulin levels and stimulating growth hormones, which ultimately work towards breaking down carbohydrates and body fat and speeding its use for energy.

Thus, Intermittent Fasting effectively tackles both sides of the calorie equation – decreasing the intake with fewer meals and increasing the burnout with an increased metabolic rate.

A 2014 scientific literature review showed a 3 – 8% weight loss over 0.75 to 6 months due to Intermittent Fasting. A loss of 4 – 7% of waist circumference was also reported, which indicates the loss of belly fat.

One such study proved that Intermittent Fasting was better compared to continuous calorie restriction as it resulted in lesser muscle loss.

2) Reduced insulin resistance and Lower risk of diabetes: There is no doubt diabetes is a serious health condition and one that has become increasingly common over the past few decades, particularly type-2 diabetes.

Type-2 diabetes occurs essentially when the body's blood sugar level rises above normal and the body has a higher insulin resistance, which means the insulin is not being used properly.

Consequently, anything that would help lower this insulin resistance should eventually contribute to lowering one's blood glucose level and prevent (or protect against) type 2 diabetes.

Intermittent Fasting, in this regard, has been proven to result in notable blood sugar level reduction.

Studies have shown that Intermittent Fasting leads to a 20 – 31% decrease in insulin resistance while decreasing the blood glucose by 3 – 6%.

Additionally, according to a study conducted on diabetic rats, Intermittent Fasting appears to protect against and prevent damage to the kidney which happens to be one of the biggest complications of diabetes.

Based on a 2014 review paper in the Translational Research journal, overweight and obese adults who observed Intermittent Fasting showed a reduction in diabetes markers i.e. insulin sensitivity.

All this implies that people at risk of becoming a victim of type-2 diabetes can use Intermittent Fasting to protect against it.

3) Improved heart health: Heart disease happens to be one of the leading causes of death in the world. Such diseases are more or less caused by the unhealthy eating habits of our generation.

Numerous risk factors are linked to increased or decreased risk of heart disease.

A 2016 review claims that Intermittent Fasting in both humans and livestock could result in reduced blood pressure, cholesterol, heart rate, and triglycerides. By the end of the day, anything unhealthy directly affects the heart and it is important to keep your heart in a healthy condition.

4) Improved brain health: Brain health is not something that should be taken lightly and efforts must be made to ensure that an individual is physically, and more importantly, mentally sound.

And Intermittent Fasting goes a long way in this regard. Metabolic features are known to be extremely important for brain health and, as previously mentioned, Intermittent Fasting has proven to improve several of these features, including a reduction in oxidative stress, inflammation, insulin resistance, and blood sugar levels – all of which are associated with neurological conditions.

Several studies conducted on mice have shown the positive results of Intermittent Fasting as it has boosted the growth of their nerve cells which has improved their brain function.

One study which compared the learning ability and memory of mice on an Intermittent Fasting diet and mice with free access to food showed that the former was better at retaining as well as acquiring new information.

Intermittent Fasting has also been known to increase brain-derived neurotrophic factor (BDNF) levels, a brain hormone the deficiency of which could lead to depression and several other neurological disorders.

Certain animal studies have discovered that the risk of neurological disorders, such as Alzheimer's disease, Parkinson's disease, Huntington's disease, and strokes can be reduced with the help of Intermittent Fasting.

5) Prevention of Alzheimer's disease: as stated above, Intermittent Fasting is beneficial for mental health but its impact on the world's most common neurogenerative diseases like Alzheimer's is even more crucial. Alzheimer's disease is an incurable condition, which means preventing it from occurring in the first place is critical.

Intermittent Fasting studies conducted on rats showed a delay in early-onset Alzheimer's and even decreased its severity.

In addition to that, a series of case reports brought to light the fact that a lifestyle intervention that included Intermittent Fasting resulted in considerable improvement in the disease's symptoms in 9 out of 10 patients.

6) Anti-aging benefits and protection against chronic diseases: one of the factors contributing to aging and chronic diseases is oxidative stress. This refers to an imbalance between the antioxidants in one's body and the free radicals.

Research carried out has shown Intermittent Fasting to boost the body's resistance to oxidative stress, thus, providing anti-aging benefits. Moreover, Intermittent Fasting helps guard against inflammation – a major cause of several common diseases.

7) Reduced risk of cancer: cancer, a terrible disease resulting from uncontrollable growth (mutation) of cells, can be prevented with Intermittent Fasting. Intermittent Fasting's effective impact on a body's metabolic rate (as discussed earlier) has been known to reduce the risk of having cancer.

Animal studies have come up with promising evidence of the prevention of cancer through Intermittent Fasting as they have shown that such restrictive diets delayed the onset of tumors in animals who observed it.

A study on human cancer patients who observed Intermittent Fasting showed a reduction in various chemotherapy side effects.

Given the fact that obesity is a major health marker for several tumors, the weight loss aspect of Intermittent Fasting could also be a contributor to the reduced risk of cancer.

Finally, Intermittent Fasting can also help prevent cancer through its effect on insulin levels and inflammation, which are among the various biological factors associated with cancer.

8) Extension of Lifespan: one of the most intriguing applications of Intermittent Fasting yet is its potential to extend the lifespan and help one live longer.

Animal researches, particularly the studies on rats, show that Intermittent Fasting contributes to lifespan extension in the same way as a continuous calorie restriction does.

One study showed a dramatic increase in lifespan by 83% in the rats which fasted compared to those who did not.

Therapeutic benefits of Intermittent Fasting

Physical benefits – Intermittent Fasting is being authenticated as an aid for preventing seizures and brain damage caused by seizures. It also gives a healing hand in curing arthritis (inflammation in joints). It also helps to reduce the toxic effects of chemotherapy and alternate-day fasting also reduces the chances of cancer.

Spiritual benefits – Fasting is known to be a spiritual practice in many religions and cultures all across the globe. All religions are different and unique, yet all of them share and promote fasting as a healing and healthy practice.

A healthy body makes the soul healthy and peaceful; this is perhaps the most important beneficial spiritual aspect. Thus, if you are looking for regaining the spirituality of your soul and bringing peace to your inner-self; Intermittent Fasting is the best of all options.

Psychological benefits – When you are fasting, you are constantly controlling your mind and are consciously choosing not to eat. This trains your brain muscles and helps them to strengthen.

After learning how to control your mind, you slowly develop the power to control further aspects of your life too. Recent studies have shown that Intermittent Fasting helped women to increase a sense of achievement, control, pride, and self-esteem.

And when you finally break your fast and enter into the feeding window; you gain an incredible sense of life, gratitude for food and nutrition, and feel blissful because of nourishment of the body.

3 Famous Intermittent Fasting schedules

There are many ways of integrating Intermittent Fasting. The three most common ones include:

Daily Intermittent Fasting – A fasting schedule that has a daily window of feeding and fasting windows. You define these windows as you want. Begin from short windows and slowly progress to large time windows.

Weekly Intermittent Fasting – A fasting schedule that requires you to specify 2 or 3 days of the week to fast. Start by fasting two days of the week, strengthen and make your body habitual and then move towards 3 days fast in a week schedule.

Alternative Day Intermittent Fasting – A fasting schedule that alternates between 24 hours of fasting and 24 hours of eating. This is not for beginners. People just getting introduced to Intermittent Fasting should not try this fasting.

It is for only those who have mastered the above two fasting schedules and are looking for a tougher challenge. These schedules are designed for individuals who want to go easy, simple, and non-complex.

Many of the readers and researchers look up for to-the-point understanding and implementation of these schedules. Therefore, precise detail is described below for each one of these schedules.

Daily Intermittent Fasting

The daily Intermittent Fasting schedule involves a 16-hour fasting period, which is then followed by an 8-hour feeding period. The 8-hour feeding window could be whatever suits one depending on their lifestyles – whether it starts from 7 am to 3 pm or from 1 pm to 9 pm.

The first and foremost consideration is the feeding window's duration. If you are just a beginner and are just stepping into the fasting lifestyle, then you should start from shorter fasting windows and longer feeding windows. For example, instead of a 16-hour fasting window, start with a 12 or 13-hour fasting window.

This will help your body to adjust to the new changes and you will not over-exhaust yourself in the very beginning. When you see that you have built-up enough stamina and can easily undergo a 12-hour fasting window, slowly increase the fasting window and move it up by one hour.

Now, you will practice this level of fasting and in this way slowly progress towards the 16/8 fasting schedule. As the name suggests, this routine is carried out every day, which makes it easier to get into the habit of a certain eating schedule.

All one needs is to learn when not to eat and the whole schedule is easily set in place. Despite the numerous pros, a possible disadvantage of the daily Intermittent Fasting model Intermittent Fasting is that since there is a 16-hour fasting window, a meal or two is easily cut out every single day.

This means the body's weekly calorie intake goes down and the observer ends up losing weight. This, depending on one's goals, could be a pro or a con – pro for someone aiming at weight loss and a con for the one trying to maintain their calorie intake.

Maintaining a chart, like the following one, could help one in sticking to an assigned schedule.

Daily Intermittent Fasting Chart

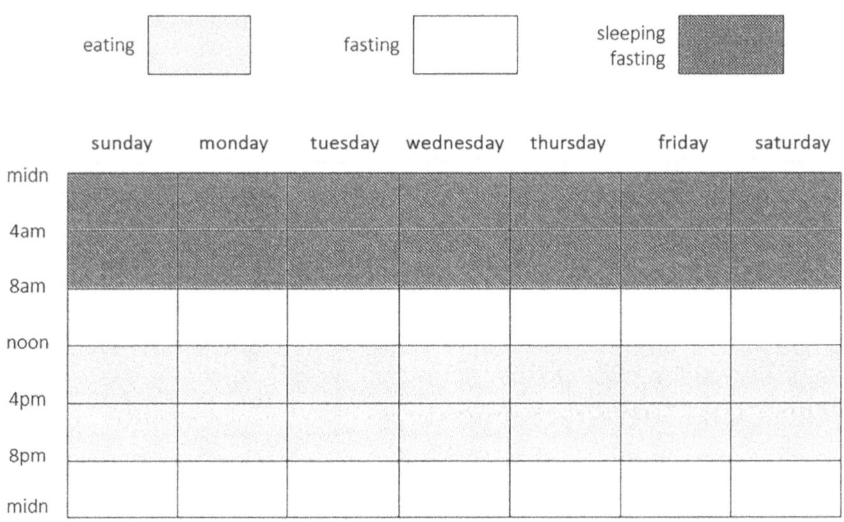

Weekly Intermittent Fasting

A preferred way to get on with Intermittent Fasting is to observe it just once every week. The weekly Intermittent Fasting has been linked to several of the benefits shared earlier in the book.

Thus, even if the goal behind using this technique is not related to weight loss or cutting down calories, this method would still yield a positive outcome.

An example of Weekly Intermittent Fasting would be to have lunch, say at midnight, on Sunday, and then fast until lunchtime on Monday. This would give a 24-hour fasting period each week.

This technique would allow one to reap the benefits of fasting while still eating every day of the week. Given the fact that only 2 meals within a weak are skipped, it is unlikely that one would lose weight.

Hence, if the objective is to lose weight, weekly intermittent would not be the best option. But if losing the calories is not an issue and the aim is to simply maintain a healthy lifestyle, then this technique is the way to go.

One of the biggest pros of weekly Intermittent Fasting is that it helps shatter the “mental barrier of fasting”.

This means that if one has never experienced fasting before, observing fasting using this technique would help one ease into it without emotionally disturbing them.

This flexible approach to intermittent fasting may be good for beginners because this may feel more natural for some people than the other fasting methods.

A sample chart, like the one below, could be used to plan out weekly Intermittent Fasting.

Weekly Intermittent Fasting Chart

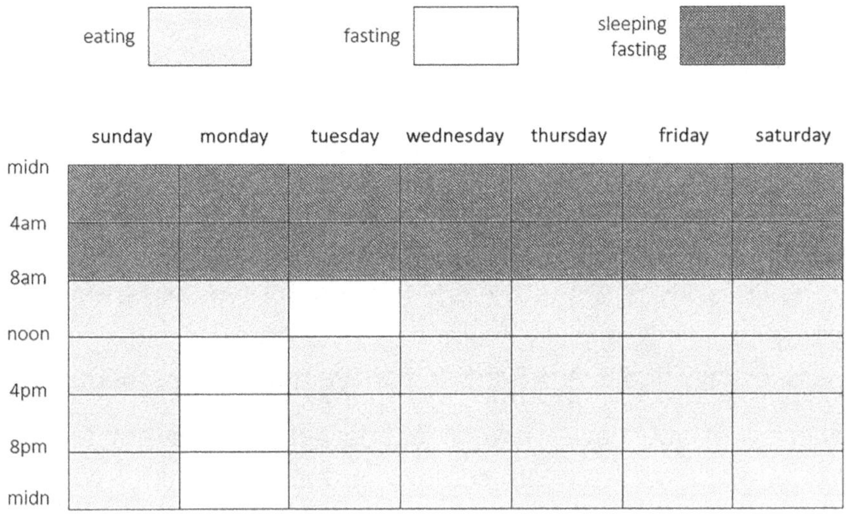

Alternate Day Intermittent Fasting

Alternate day Intermittent Fasting, as the name suggests, refers to longer fasting windows on alternate days in a week. In alternate day Intermittent Fasting, for instance, if one eats dinner on Sunday, he or she would then fast for 24 hours and have their next meal on Monday evening.

Tuesday would be a feeding period and one would eat all day and then start the next 24-hour fasting cycle after having dinner on Tuesday evening, and so on. This method allows one to have at least one meal per day and still enjoy the benefits of long fasting periods consistently. As you can see; this fasting schedule is harder and longer than all others. In this fasting schedule, you have to stay on a fast for 24 hours, and then for the next 24 hours, you can eat.

This is not best suitable for beginners. This can prove extremely hard for you if you are just stepping into the fasting world. Always make sure to start easy and slowly progress your way to the top.

An advantage of alternate day Intermittent Fasting is that it increases the benefits of fasting, hypothetically, compared to daily Intermittent Fasting because it involves having longer fasted state time as compared to the latter. Practically, however, it is not as suitable. This method makes it extremely difficult to have enough feast days to make up for the fasted days.

This way of Intermittent Fasting is, therefore, not too common in the real world and is mostly used by bodybuilders and professionals who can take easily take up this type of fasting. The general public especially women with already sensitive insulin levels, usually find it very hard to manage this fasting schedule.

Especially if you have irregular eating patterns, do not try this schedule at first. Start with something that is doable for you and once you get comfortable with that, you can increase the fasting or feeding window and move on. The chart below is an example of Alternate Day Intermittent Fasting.

Alternate Day Intermittent Fasting Chart

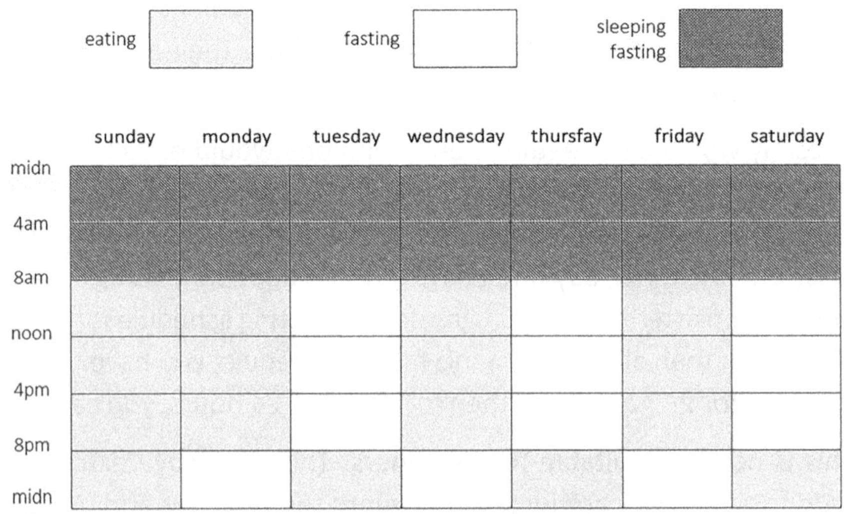

Note:

The best option is to try and incorporate daily and weekly Intermittent Fasting styles. Start-off with a weekly fasting schedule which requires you to fast two days a week.

Once you are comfortable with the weekly schedule, progress your way to daily fasting.

Practice observing it once a week or once a month and then decide for yourself, which of these IF schedules suit you the best.

Strategies of IF that proved most beneficial for women

There are many techniques and methods out there for Intermittent Fasting. But it is important to note that not every one of them is suitable for women.

Some require extreme and drastic measures like staying hungry for extraordinarily long periods. This can disturb the diet plan for women and also might disturb the hormonal balance and may start hundreds of other problems.

Some types of Intermittent Fasting are specifically designed for bodybuilders and men. Following those types can severely impact the health of women because they are too tough to implement. That is why; the types of Intermittent Fasting that have been proven beneficial for women are listed below:

1) The 5:2 Intermittent Fasting:

The 5:2 fasting method is the most popular and most common Intermittent Fasting method. It is called the '5:2' because you eat 5 days of the week in a normal and regular pattern.

While the remaining two days of the week, you limit your calorie intake. The limit is between 500 to 600 calories per day.

Again, it is not a diet, so you are not restricted on what to eat and what to avoid. You can choose anything that you want to eat, you just have to limit it's intake to a fixed number of calories.

Meaning eating small portions at one time and increase the number of meals if you want to. It all depends on you; you are the one in the driving seat and can make decisions according to your routine and work schedule.

How to implement this method? First of all, think about your schedule and the busiest days of the week. You can opt not to fast on those days so that it doesn't pressure you or your diet.

So, choose the 5 days you don't want to fast on and eat regularly as you used to on those days. Then, pick two days on which you can fast easily and they should have an average gap between them.

For example, if you are choosing Tuesday as day one of your fast, then pick Friday as the second day. This will allow an even gap between your fast which is a gap of three days between each fasting day. Whatever days you choose, there must be at least one or two-day gap between them.

After choosing your fasting days, suiting your lifestyle and routine, the second step is to think of dividing your calorie intake for your days of fasting.

Meaning that since you have 500 calorie intake allowed, divide them into two meals of 250 calories or you can increase the number of meals by further shrinking the size of the meal.

This will keep you active and energized throughout the day besides the fact that you are fasting.

Do not take one meal of 500 calories because after 8 to 12 hours you will feel hunger levels striking very high and you will be unable to eat anything since you have already consumed your calorie intake of the day. This will leave you lethargic and lazy for the rest of the day.

So, either you can have three small meals consisting of breakfast, lunch, and dinner. Or have two slightly bigger meals; lunch and dinner only.

It is normal to feel hungry and weaker on the first few fasts, but your body will very soon adjust to new changes and you will get used to fast days and won't affect you that much.

In conclusion, this is a type of intermittent fast that you can customize according to yourself. Every woman can fix the days suiting her and her schedule and thus every woman out there can benefit from this method of fasting.

How is it beneficial for women? 5:2 is extremely easy and simple to implement. Every woman can tailor this fasting method according to herself. Women with kids and work can choose differently and housewives can choose differently.

It provides you the flexibility that no other diet will ever provide you. It spares you from tedious calculations of daily calorie intake. It does not prohibit you from eating your favorite foods.

The only condition is to not go overboard with them and amalgamate healthy and nutritious foods in your diet too.

So, your body keeps receiving the necessary nutrition supply and you can lose weight without losing patience or health.

Advantages:

- You don't have to follow calorie restrictions every day, thus making it easier to implement.
- Many studies have shown that regular calorie restriction helps to lose weight more efficiently.

- Women with higher insulin levels can benefit from it because this fasting method lowers the insulin levels in the body.
- It also improves insulin sensitivity.
- It reduces fat mass without affecting muscle mass.
- It also helps to reduce weight as well as inflammation in bodies.

2) Intermittent Fasting with 8-hour Eating Window:

If you follow an 8-hour eating window fasting, it means that your fasting window is of 16 hours and your feeding window is of 8 hours. It is also one of the simplest and easiest fasting methods and beneficial for women since it doesn't require full days of fasting.

It just needs specifying which portion of the day to fast and in which portion to eat.

This is also an adaptable and adjustable fasting way and anyone can fix the hours according to their lifestyle and schedule. The most common practice followed by the practitioners of this technique is fast from dinner to lunch.

This only makes you skip breakfast and you also complete the fasting window without stressing your body too much. The key point of this fasting method is Consistency.

If you do not follow the same schedule every day, staying hungry for 16 hours won't matter. The reason being you are not training your body to burn incessantly present fats inside the body.

The body won't be able to learn your eating habits and thus it won't be able to make a decision when to burn the fats and when not to.

It is because you are eating at inconsistent hours and are constantly changing your fasting and feeding windows.

Some women like to keep light exercising in their daily schedule. Strict diet plans followed with exercise is too much exhaustion for women's bodies.

Therefore, this Intermittent Fasting technique helps women to maintain a fasting schedule, maintain a healthy and nutritious feeding schedule, and also incorporate light exercising.

Many women have reported that this technique has worked the best for them and they never stopped following it because of its excellent results in weight loss while maintaining a healthy body.

Those who are looking for how to start Intermittent Fasting are suggested to start by implementing this fasting method. It is the simplest and requires the least effort on the practitioner's end.

It is not an extreme food deprivation technique, thus making it easy for beginners to enter a healthy lifestyle.

How to implement this method? Simply select the 16-hour fasting window and 8-hour feeding window. This selection is based solely on your lifestyle and work schedule.

If you have tough and tedious working hours during the day then choose the evening and night as your fasting window.

And if you are a beginner and are looking for the easiest way to start Intermittent Fasting, choose windows that make you skip breakfast. That way you can enjoy lunch and dinner and fast through the night. Again, this method is customizable according to anyone.

How is it beneficial for women? Women with extremely hard days and having busiest schedules are suggested to start from a 14-hour fasting window and a 10-hour feeding window.

This might seem more doable and more practical to women since they have lower energy levels than men. Once you are comfortable with the 14:10 hour window, move towards the 16:8 hour window.

This is a huge convenience for women since they can start slow and move further along according to their pace and stamina.

Many other fasting ways like 24-hour fasting is not suitable for women.

This technique is inspired by bodybuilders and weight-lifters. Since it requires extreme deprivation of food for 24 hours and then heavy and full of protein meals for the next 24 hours helps bodybuilders to achieve higher body mass and muscles.

Women cannot benefit from this technique at all. It may disturb their eating and sleeping schedules. That's why; 8-hour feeding Intermittent Fasting is extremely beneficial for women.

Advantages:

- Start according to your own pace and stamina.
- The best way of Intermittent Fasting for beginners.
- Customizable for every individual.
- Easy and simple to implement.
- No need for keeping track of calorie intake all the time.
- Saves busy women a lot of time and effort.
- Once the beginner level is achieved, you can move to even longer fasting windows.
- Gives time to your body to adapt to the fasting schedule.
- Doesn't leave you feeling weak or low in energy.

3) Spontaneously skip the meals:

This is a non-scheduled type of fasting unlike the above-mentioned ways of fasting. While other ways of Intermittent Fasting require a schedule keeping and keeping track of fasting and feeding windows, this type of fasting is conducted whenever convenient.

For example, women who are free on weekends and don't have much activity these days can skip meals when they are not feeling hungry. Because your activity is lessened on the weekend, it is quite appropriate to lessen your food intake too.

This will automatically reduce the calorie count inside your body and you will lose weight without even trying. Skipping a meal or two spontaneously is also an intermittent fast.

Though spontaneous and unplanned, yet it benefits you the same way as a planned fast would. Suppose you are traveling and haven't found a healthy food spot, start a fast.

And then when you reach your destination, you would already have burned a lot of fat and then by eating healthy foods, you will supply the nutrition to your body without giving it access to calories.

Spontaneous fasting has proven very beneficial in many kinds of research and studies. The human body is well-equipped to handle long periods of hunger and fasting because this starts up the process of disintegration of stored body fats.

When you skip a meal, your body doesn't get a resource of energy from outside.

That's what forces it to decompose existing fat residing inside the fat cells. This is a very healthy approach towards weight loss and anyone can do it anytime, anywhere.

How is it beneficial for women? Have you been working all day and couldn't find time to prepare a meal and to eat it? You just performed a spontaneous intermittent fast!

How does this help you? Your body has been taking its necessary fuel from fat reservoirs inside your body and unconsciously you have lost a bunch of calories.

Your body practiced how to depend on its own-self in a case when you skip a meal and next time when you skip a meal; it knows how to refuel the energy tank. Thus, unknowingly and without trying you removed some of the access from your body.

Advantages:

- Triggers the present at the inside body.
- Burns the excess fat presiding in fat cells.
- Provides energy to your body while shedding off extra fat.
- No need of following schedules of eating and fasting.
- Unplanned and easy weight loss.

4) Reducing portions of food during the 'Feeding-Window':

This is an Intermittent Fasting technique that is implemented very slowly and steadily. This technique also doesn't require following any schedules. It just demands slowly reducing food portions when you are eating during your feeding-window.

This is an automatic technique of fasting; meaning by slowly reducing the daily calorie intake, you automatically come under the Intermittent Fasting technique.

It resembles the '5:2 Intermittent Fasting' because you limit your calorie intake during the fasting days. The difference is; you don't have to define the fasting days.

Just simply reduce calorie intake and you won't need to maintain schedules of fasting and non-fasting.

How to implement this method? The goal is to take your diet towards smaller meal portions. But the key point is to not be rash and extra fast while doing so. This might leave the body dealing and coping with deficiencies.

Therefore, be slow and gentle while doing so. Start by lessening the portion a tiny bit and work your way up to eating small portions of food and still satisfy your appetite.

How is this beneficial for women? While the majority of the women out there and already tired and fed-up from stupid and lame dieting which hasn't worked out for them.

And they have ended up gaining the lost weight in no time. Those women are done following any strict eating schedules and diet plans and are thus looking for some natural ways to lose weight.

This way of Intermittent Fasting brings ease to them because they do not have to put any extra effort or follow strict eating schedules.

They just have to slowly pace their appetite and move towards shorter portions of the meal. This will automatically bring the body into the habit of eating less and moving more thus enabling you to lose extra pounds without struggling.

Advantages:

- Convenient and simple.
- Slower than other techniques yet more beneficial.
- Losing weight without extreme dieting and exercising.
- Less calorie intake, a higher possibility of weight loss.

How to get started with Intermittent Fasting?

Since now you have the information about what are the different ways and strategies for Intermittent Fasting, all you have to do now is to choose one method and implement it.

The easiest way to get started is to pick a method that sounds easy to you and you think you will be able to pull-off. Begin it from there; see how it affects your overall health and energy.

It is true that in the start you will feel a little weak but observe for longer patterns, if you do re-gain your energy levels even after implementing the fasting then keep ongoing.

If the method is not suiting you or your body in any way, then you can stop and move on towards another strategy. Intermittent Fasting has a learning curve attached to it.

It will take you some time to get habitual and understand what your body is telling you. You might not get it on the first try; you might have to browse through different ways and techniques of Intermittent Fasting to get it right.

Keep on implementing the strategies until you find the best suitable fasting schedule. Also, you don't necessarily have to follow a well-structured plan for Intermittent Fasting.

As discussed before, some Intermittent Fasting strategies don't require any strict schedule-following or calorie-counting.

If you are a busy person and don't have much time to focus on the details then simply go for spontaneous fasting or random fasting days.

Even the strategy of making your meals small might do the job for you. It just needs some time to familiarize yourself with Intermittent Fasting and how it works.

In conclusion, if you are looking for pointers on how to start with Intermittent Fasting, you can go ahead and read the 7-Day Beginner's Guide for Intermittent Fasting.

It has all the possible help and tips listed and you will not need much guidance after reading it.

It has taken into account every possible consideration for beginners and has been made easy so that everyone feels welcomed and comfortable in beginning with an Intermittent Fasting lifestyle.

Intermittent fasting can provide significant health benefits if it is done right, with perseverance and without overdoing it. Of course, in this case, time works for us.

Anyway, Intermittent Fasting may not be for you if you have an eating disorder, are pregnant or breastfeeding, have diabetes, are taking certain medications, or are under 18 years old.

Consult with your physician if you have any of these conditions before trying IF.

Chapter 3

Design your own IF program

Intermittent Fasting offers many programs and it is still possible that you don't find any of the described programs suitable for you.

Fortunately, Intermittent Fasting extends the facility and ease of designing your very own program. You can choose your day too fast as well as your feeding and fasting window and you might be wanting to have just a few exceptions in your Intermittent Fasting program.

Must Note!

Designing your Intermittent Fasting program is not recommended for beginners. You must first try some authentic Intermittent Fasting programs and experiment with them before moving on to defining your own. If you don't have any experience with Intermittent Fasting before, then while creating your program you may go wrong somewhere and might also make mistakes that may impact your health and body.

So initially, follow a recognized Intermittent Fasting program, follow its directions, and then after experimentation with different Intermittent Fasting programs you find none of them are suitable for you, you can move on to designing one of your own.

That way, you will have some helpful pointers and experience that will guide you on how to get the best out of Intermittent Fasting.

Helpful pointers for designing your own IF program: You will notice that all the Intermittent Fasting programs have a few common things. These commonalities can act as your reference guide and can provide you a general guideline on how to design your Intermittent Fasting program.

A few of the commonalities are listed below for your ease:

- The fasting period is generally longer than the feeding period.

- All IF programs have a 'feeding state' and a 'fed state'.
- In none of the programs, the fasting window exceeds 24 hours. So, make sure, do not design a fasted state comprising of more than 24 hours because in that case it will be called 'starvation' and not 'fasting'.

How to design your own IF program? Researches have shown that many women frequently ask questions about how to design a successful Intermittent Fasting program, what things to include, and what things to avoid. So, here is a general explanation of the guidelines that you should follow to design a completely healthy and successful IF program.

1) **Decide how often would you like to fast?** Would you prefer it doing daily, weekly, or every other day? This decision is solely based on your work schedule, your lifestyle, and your will to lose weight. If you want great results and you are very serious about losing weight then you might lean towards daily fasting. It is slightly hard but very efficient. And if you are just casually exploring different types of fasting and do not want to lose too much too fast then you may incline towards a weekly schedule where you just need to fast one or two days a week. So, first of all, decide how often you would like to fast depending on your preferences.
2) **Decide how long can you fast?** If you are just entering the Intermittent Fasting world, then you should choose shorter fasting periods. But if you have a few month's experience with Intermittent Fasting, then you can opt for longer periods of fasting. This all depends on your stamina, your willpower, and your health condition. People with higher stamina and better health can go for long fasts, but people with low stamina and already low energy levels should try short fasts. Spontaneous fasts can also help you in this

regard. Thus, decide how long you can fast and it should not exceed 24 hours!

3) **Decide what you want to eat during your feeding window?** Are you thinking about why this is important? It is important because if you just had a sandwich in your feeding window, then it is likely that you will get hungry again much faster and thus your next fasting window will have to be short. But if you had a big and healthy meal after your fast, then you can go for a longer duration of fasting the next time. Remember that eating healthy during your feeding state is important and your body will benefit from it. It might even heal your body and provide strengthening nutrition to your body.
4) **Put your plan in the execution phase!** Now that you have figured out what to do and when to do it, you can now put your plan into action. It is better if you start your Intermittent Fasting program the very next day or week depending on which type of Intermittent Fasting you chose. If you keep on delaying it onto the next day or next week, you will never be able to start. Do it and do it now! If you keep on postponing it, and anxiety will keep on building inside your mind and that anxiety might lead you towards fear of starting. Plan well and start immediately. This will spare you all the drama and anxiety and might even help you to feel enthusiastic about this experience.

Protocols necessary to succeed in Intermittent Fasting

Although Intermittent Fasting is itself a well-rounded technique and doesn't require extreme measures to be taken to succeed.

Still, some factors contribute to its success factors and some protocols need to be followed to get the best possible results in a shorter time. You can adjust the eating and fasting windows; you can choose the fasting days according to your will but there are a few necessary guidelines you need to know. Listed below are some important protocols to keep in mind to achieve a 100% success rate through Intermittent Fasting:

Food quality. One of the most important factors that contribute to the success of Intermittent Fasting is food quality. If you have been fasting and then you satisfy your appetite with junk food or unhealthy food every time; your body will not receive the necessary nutrients and proteins.

This will leave a negative impact on your body; more importantly on your health. Intermittent Fasting doesn't restrict you to specific foods but it does recommend eating healthy. Intermittent Fasting doesn't prohibit you from eating what you like but it does require a balance in the diet. If you had a burger or pizza for lunch, have something healthy for dinner. The quality of the food matters too.

Don't keep eating old food. Have a fresh meal every time. This will help you feel healthier and more energized.

Consistency. The second but important factor is '*Consistency*'. Just like all other dieting plans, Intermittent Fasting also requires its practitioner to be consistent. You might not get the best results soon, but remain consistent and keep following the strategy for longer periods for it to work.

It's possible that at first, you might feel the urge to quit, but research shows that women who stuck with it for extended periods were the ones happiest from its results.

So, after you pick out an Intermittent Fasting strategy or schedule, stick with it and hold on to it, and don't lose consistency.

It's a famous quote that 'good things take time' and it is 100% true while following Intermittent Fasting. Never lose hope or get disappointed if you don't see results instantly. Just believe and keep going on until you hit your goal weight.

Calories. Indeed, Intermittent Fasting doesn't put an extremely harsh restriction on calorie count; still, the calories do matter. If you fast for some hours and then relish a heavy meal with thousands of calories, you didn't do yourself any favors. Eating "normally" is the key here.

This means that when you are in the non-fasting phase; don't try to make up for the lost calories by eating huge meals. Eat normally as you would even if you hadn't been fasting.

Some people believe that since they stayed hungry for a longer duration, high-calorie intake won't affect them since they lost so much already.

It is not at all true. Yes, you have lost a good number of calories when you were fasting, but it does not mean you can eat more than you need or more than your appetite. Maintain a balanced diet although you were fasting or not. This will help you lose more calories and gain less.

Patience. Studies have shown that many impatient people tried Intermittent Fasting and gave it up after a few weeks or a month. Just because they didn't see distinguished results in a short time, they decided to leave the practice altogether. This is not right.

Once you get into something; be patient and wait for it to work, especially when you are guaranteed that you will see the results. It can take longer than you thought.

Just be patient and keep giving complete dedication to it. It is also a fact that Intermittent Fasting takes longer than any of the crash-diets or extreme dieting plans. But it is also true that Intermittent Fasting takes a more natural approach towards losing weight.

Diets might give you results sooner than Intermittent Fasting but be assured that you must have left some nutritional deficiencies in your body that you might not be able to catch up with later. In the long run, diets have put people to bed because it insinuates hundreds of types of diseases.

Intermittent Fasting on the other hand; works naturally, doesn't ask for drastic changes, doesn't limit you to specific foods, and recommends you to eat everything in a healthy and proper amount.

So, it might take longer than dieting plans, just be patient and keep following the instructions with complete faith and be rest assured that you will lose weight and make your body healthier.

Training. There can be two types of training protocols – strength training and general learning training.

- General learning training includes familiarizing with yourself how Intermittent Fasting works, what are different strategies to implement, and learning which implementation strategy works best for you. Since you have to test out different techniques and it has a learning curve attached to it; that is why it is called general learning training.
- Strength training means training your body to lose most of your body fat while holding onto muscle weight. Women who are at a healthy weight already and they just want to stay at their goal weight without losing muscle mass lean towards this training. To not get extremely skinny and look slim; strength training is provided. In this training, you learn to keep on your muscle mass and just lose the extra fats and calories. This is very important regarding the health of your body because you never want to go overboard with fasting and become extremely weak. A good shape of the body needs muscle mass and muscle strength, and to maintain a good and appealing shape of the body, understanding and implementing strength training is important.

Significance of fluids during Intermittent Fasting

Fasting windows don't allow any food intake, but researches have proven that drinking water and non-sugary fluids speed along the process of weight loss from fasting. Keep yourself hydrated and use calorie-free drinks for the purpose. You can drink as much water as you want, both normal and sparkling, unsweetened tea, lemon water, and black coffee, because, during Intermittent Fasting, water is the best choice. But if you are not in the mood for plain water, just add a simple mint or lemon for flavor.

You are allowed to have coffee and unsweetened tea also, but remember nothing works as best as water.

Why is water important? Drinking plenty of water is not only beneficial for keeping your body hydrated but there are many other numerous health benefits too. One, water carries oxygen and other healthy nutrients and leads them to your body cells, which helps in strengthening of the body cells.

Second, it helps maintain healthy blood pressure. Third, it keeps your body temperature regular. Fourth, it keeps your digestive system healthy and regular. Fifth, it keeps your joints lubricated and strengthened. Therefore, during fasting when you are denying food from your body, it is necessary to provide nourishment to your body by drinking plenty of water.

Some people don't realize its significance and its vital role in your health and that water deficiency later takes on a horrific shape for you in the form of chronic disease.

What else can you drink?

- **Black Coffee** doesn't take you out of your fasting cycle. And many published reports imply that caffeine can boost your metabolism and this also plays a role in losing weight. But it must remain simple black coffee; any added sweeteners or cream/milk can take you right out of your fasting cycle.

- **Tea** that is free from added sugars is also beneficial during Intermittent Fasting. It not only helps in cellular detoxification but also induces probiotic balance. Although you can have all types of tea during your fast like green, black or herbal. But green tea specifically has proven to be more advantageous than other forms. It suppresses the levels of appetite and also speeds the process of weight loss.
- **Apple Cider Vinegar** can also be kept underuse during an intermittent fast. It helps in the regulation of your blood sugar and also improves digestion. That's why it might enhance the effects of Intermittent Fasting.

Drinks to avoid during Intermittent Fasting. Many zero-calorie beverages are available in the market, which is full of calories. And intentionally or unintentionally, such beverages can put you out of your fasting cycle and can knock your body out of the fasted state. Such drinks include diet soda, coconut water, sugar-free juices, alcohol, and almond milk.

Diet sodas claim that they are technically free of any calories, but it is all untrue. The artificial sweeteners added are worse than normal soda because they spike-up your insulin levels and also wreck your blood sugar levels.

Also, coconut water and almond milk might sound like they are free of sugar but they are not. Consuming these will increase your carb intake and you will eventually be put out of your fasted state. The same goes for alcohol.

Why avoiding sugary drinks is important during IF? Drinking sugary beverages initially spikes your blood sugar, after that your body goes through a dramatic drop of sugar level and this prompts your body to eat more to bring back your sugar levels to normal.

As a result, you are unable to withstand fasting since your body needs to regain sugar levels. And that's how the majority of people lose their fast cycle and immediately are out of Intermittent Fasting.

High sugar levels also prove to be addictive to your body and that's why you feel a craving again and again in your brain.

Once you have a sugary beverage, next time when you fast your body will go into a low sugar level state and it will intensely demand from you the sugar-high that you gained from the sugary beverage.

This will make it harder for you to resist eating, might even annoy you, and might create a bad impression of fasting.

Take-away. Healthy beverages like water help you to overcome some common fasting concerns. It helps in curing headaches, dizziness, constipation, and also muscle cramps. Hence, drinking plenty of fluids during fasting is extremely important.

Also, consuming sugar-free and carbs-free fluids will help you maintain a healthy fasting cycle and as a result, you will lose weight much faster and more efficiently. Beware of market claimed sugar-free products and always remember, any product that claims to be sugar-free must do something to make them taste good.

That can sometimes include artificial flavors, unnatural sweeteners, or even some chemicals. Therefore, always tend to go towards natural and healthy beverages like water.

Helpful tips for Intermittent Fasting

Always start slow. Before starting any diet or exercise or even fasting, always begin from the lowest level. Initially, you know that you are putting your body to go through a change and your body isn't prepared for it. Human bodies adapt and change with time and practice. You cannot expect that you fasted one day and the very next time you fast your body will be getting into a habit of fasting. NO! Each body takes its own time to adjust and adapt to new changes and challenges put in front of it. Intermittent Fasting offers beginner level as well as advanced levels. Beginner levels include the 8-hour eating window method and reducing meal portions.

Advanced levels include alternate day fasting in which you fast straight for 24 hours and alternate the days of fasting. It is mere stupidity to start from advanced levels. This will create thousands of deficiencies in your body because you didn't give time to the body to adjust to new changes and might end up with a chronic disease one day due to the un-fulfillment of necessary nutrition.

Therefore, start from the easiest level and progress your way to the top. Allow your body to adjust to new changes and focus on keeping a healthy nutrition

Experiment and learn. Intermittent Fasting demands a certain level of experimentation from its practitioners. Some women might think that they can start with daily Intermittent Fasting but as they start, they begin to realize it is getting tough for them.

Now, this was an experiment that didn't give them the best results or didn't prove what they hoped for. What they should do is; start spontaneous fasting. This will prepare the body to be more ready when and if you fast.

So, you performed an experiment, deduced the results, and learned what technique is best for you and what strategy suits you the best. That is why; Intermittent Fasting is called an experiment and learning technique.

Listen to your body. Human bodies are designed to adjust to new changes and with time get adapted to the changes and become habitual of them. Human bodies are embedded with the ability to send out warning signals to the brain if something is getting too exhausting and tough for the body. For example, people under chronic stress begin to have constant headaches. The headaches are a sign from the body that the stress you are going through is too much for your body and you need to relax and calm your nerves. Similarly, when you start with Intermittent Fasting, the body initially will give you signals of weakness or even dizziness.

These initial symptoms happen and there is nothing to worry about. Just give time to your body to adjust. Intermittent Fasting demands time, and if after several months of fasting, still, your body is giving signals of fatigue and low energy, it means that you are doing too much or your body is unable to cope with the loss of energy.

It is also possible that after you have started Intermittent Fasting, in a month or so your body gets completely adapted and used to the new eating schedule.

Therefore, after passing the initial stages of fasting, keep an ear on what your body is telling you. If you feel fit and healthy even after fasting that means your body is in a healthy condition.

But if you keep feeling dizziness or laziness, this might be a signal from your body that it's getting too much. Remember to always listen to what your body is telling you.

Slow and steady wins the race. Start-off at the beginner level and progress your way to harder and advanced levels of Intermittent Fasting. It works best if you keep moving slowly and steadily.

Do not act rashly and jump towards the hardest levels of Intermittent Fasting. This will snatch away the adjusting and coping period from your body and this will leave you with a hundred kinds of nutritional deficiencies or even some kind of diseases.

Pick an Intermittent Fasting schedule, stick to it for months, and then see the results and decide if the schedule has worked out for you. Don't expect extremely fast results. Intermittent Fasting is a natural way to reduce weight and that is the reason why you need to go slowly and steadily and remain consistent.

Write a journal or a make chart about your progress. Writing a journal or making a chart will help you track your progress and will help you in remembering what problems you faced.

You can start by entering your initial weight and then after every week or every month, you can update it with your current weight and mention the weight-loss. Start by making a column called the first week and enter all the information related to your first week in Intermittent Fasting. If you faced any dizziness or light-headedness, mention it down and see after how long these signs vanish.

If they vanish after a week or 10 days then be satisfied and know that you are on the right track. If they don't go away, it means that your body is trying to tell you something. If you keep on recording the intensity of these signs, it will help you to diagnose what is the root cause of this problem.

You can also write about your daily food experience. One day if you enjoy a slightly heavier meal and the next day you just eat some veggies, then it will be beneficial for you to compare the results and see which day you felt better.

If heavy meals made you feel lazy and less energetic then you can have helpful pointers on how to avoid it from happening again.

You can track the patterns of eating; see how different foods affect your health and activity of the day. At the end of the day, you can decide for yourself if you are progressing or if Intermittent Fasting is not suitable for you.

Be more active and productive. It is a common perception that when you are fasting, you should rest and not move around much since your body is going through a fasting window.

This perception is not healthy and doesn't work out for the best. Remember, always act "normal"; doesn't matter if you are fasting or not. "Acting normal" means continue to be active throughout the day, eat in the same way if you weren't having been fasting and this is the way to precisely train the body to get used to the new Intermittent Fasting schedule.

If you think that fasting and getting plenty of rest and eating a heavy meal afterward is necessary to make up for lost energy then you couldn't have been more wrong. The main purpose of Intermittent Fasting is to enable individuals to fast and lose weight naturally.

That means to continue with daily jobs and activities as if you are not fasting. Staying active and productive will keep your body in a healthy and active state and will keep you energized throughout the day.

During the eating windows; choose nutritious foods. After completing the 'fasted window' when you enter the 'feeding window', always keep in mind to eat as if you were not on a fast and it is just another normal meal of the day.

Also, your body needs necessary nutrients like protein and iron, so you must include healthy items on your menu. This will help restore the nutrition of the body and will keep you energized enough for further fast days.

If you relish an unhealthy and heavy meal after a fast, it will slow down your metabolism and create tons of digestive problems. So, maintaining a healthy diet is very crucial for the success of Intermittent Fasting.

Eat everything but in small portions. The best thing about Intermittent Fasting is that it does not limit your food choices.

Unlike diets, which limit you to only a few foods, Intermittent Fasting doesn't restrict you in this regard. You can eat anything you wish to eat. The only condition is to maintain a balance.

That is, if you ate a heavy meal at one time then you should eat something very light and healthy in the next meal.

Don't restrict what you eat, just limit everything you eat. Eating relatively smaller portions of meals each day will automatically train your digestive system and metabolism to stay active and work at their best in the given conditions.

Thus, you will not be forced to abstain from foods you love, every once in a while, you can have whatever you want to eat.

Intermittent Fasting is a convenience; not a strict obligation. Dieting plans are designed to be strict and put limitations on your overall eating habits. Dieting forces you to keep eating one type of food; for example, low-calorie foods.

Dieting restricts you to eat very less after huge intervals of starvation. There is no wiggling room according to each individual. There are strict rules that everyone has to follow. This is where Intermittent Fasting comes in.

It provides you a much convenient option than dieting. You can choose your fasting schedule; you can choose whatever you want to eat and you also get to choose when to eat it.

Intermittent Fasting allows you to define your own fasted and fed states and this allows every individual to feel comfortable and convenient with this weight-loss method.

Therefore; people who enjoy a restriction-free lifestyle and want to be in charge of their eating habits, lean much more towards Intermittent Fasting rather than conventional dieting methods.

Intermittent Fasting provides a comfortable, convenient, flexible way for women who want to lose weight while enjoying their life and keeping their bodies healthy.

How to use Intermittent Fasting for muscle gain?

The most negative and the worst side-effect of dieting is that body burns muscle along with fats. This side-effect takes a strong negative toll on your health. Instead of losing excess fats, you start to lose your muscle which makes you weak from inside.

Dieting has strict calorie restrictions and after losing fat it induces the loss of muscle inside the body.

Many research studies have been conducted in this regard and it has been proven that Intermittent Fasting interestingly lets you hold on to muscle while burning fat.

The researches have shown that dieting induces a 25% reduction in muscle mass and this is catastrophic in the long term.

That's why Intermittent Fasting is extremely beneficial for women who are trying to hold on to their muscle mass and just shed-off the extra pounds they have gained.

How to gain muscle during IF? If you are working out while fasting side by side, you are more likely to burn more fat while sustaining muscle. Insulin sensitivity is the relation between the two.

If you are decreasing your calorie intake during your feeding window then you will burn higher fat in your fasting window.

This means that when you consume food it is distributed how it should be. It will take place of the lost energy and will leave your muscle mass alone. People are always looking to hear the good news that the food you eat serves the right purpose.

So Intermittent Fasting gives this good news to the people who are looking to lose fat while keeping muscles intact. The quality of the food you consume during your 'feeding window' decides the muscle growth and weight loss.

If you are constantly consuming low-quality foods then you will lose the strength of the muscles eventually.

Weight loss is a must when you fast, but if you want to gain muscle while doing so; you must increase the quality of the food you are eating. It should be healthy and nutritious so that weight-loss doesn't draw out muscle mass too.

Tips for gaining muscle during Intermittent Fasting:

- If you are looking to increase your muscle gain, then you don't need to worry about meal timings too much. Just keep fasting and feeding regularly and you will see that you will lose weight while keeping your muscle mass intact.
- Don't be afraid of calorie-restrictions. After fasting, you can enjoy a healthy and moderate-sized meal. You shouldn't worry about only eating low-calorie foods and restricting your meal portions. Eat freely to satisfy your diet.
- Do not restrict yourself from different kinds of foods. Integrate all kinds of foods in your diet, because you never know what food helps you the most to lose weight while incessantly gaining muscle mass.
- Simply changing your meal timings can significantly promote muscle growth. When you only eat at restricted timings every day, you will only lose weight and it won't affect your muscle growth. So, keep on changing the time of your meals and see what timing best suits your muscle growth.
- When we fast our insulin, levels drop and it helps to burn the fat, when we eat our insulin levels increase and helps to restore the energy of the body. Therefore, keeping an abstaining attitude from calories will help you lose weight, but it won't help you in increasing your muscle growth. So,

during your feeding window, don't feel restricted from what to eat and what not to eat. Eat freely and eat healthily.

Common mistakes to avoid during Intermittent Fasting

Many people start with Intermittent Fasting with high hope, but because of some conscious or unconscious mistakes, they have a bad experience with it. These mistakes might hinder in the way of effective weight-loss, overall satisfaction, and ease of the process.

Below listed are a few of the most common mistakes that are observed way too many times. So, providing information about them and highlight the ways to avoid them is important.

Giving up too early. Any weight-loss program is hard. Either it is dieting or workout exercises or even Intermittent Fasting. You are keeping yourself in a fasting state and that means you have to avoid eating food for several hours. This is not easy to do at first. Your body is in a habit of receiving continuous nutrition.

And then when you start to fast, you are stopping the nutrition supply. So of course, you are going to face difficulty in the initial stages of fasting. You will experience feelings of exhaustion and irritability.

But be assured that these feelings will go away after a week or two. Just be patient and wait for these symptoms to go away.

Once your body gets used to the new schedules, you will feel much more energetic and healthier. And you will start to appreciate Intermittent Fasting.

The main point here is not to give up too early. Everything demands time. It is also quite possible that the fasting method you chose doesn't fit quite well with your lifestyle.

So, don't hurry and throw in the towel too soon. Just hold on patiently and experiment with different types of fasting methods and see what works best for you. Rashly deciding that fasting is not suitable for you and give it up too quickly is one of the biggest mistakes that people make.

You must know that Intermittent Fasting needs you to be calm, steady, and patient. Results of Intermittent Fasting also can take longer than any other dieting plans, but the wait will be worth it.

Making drastic changes in your eating patterns. Too much change too suddenly can have negative impacts instead of positive ones.

If normally you eat after every 3 to 4 hours and then suddenly one day shrink the eating window of the entire day to an 8-hour window, then this might be a too drastic change for your body.

You will be left feeling discouraged and hungry all the time. This is one of the biggest reasons that make people quit fasting.

Each body needs time to adjust to new changes and everyone has a different adjusting time.

The quote 'slow and steady wins the race' works best in this situation. If you suddenly start from a 14 or 16 hour fast, your body won't be able to catch-up to such drastic changes.

It may take you a week or 10 days to adjust to new schedules and long fasting windows. Gradually stretch out the number of hours between each meal and once you reach a 10 or 12-hour gap between your meals, then start a regular and strict fasting schedule.

Because then your body will be ready to take the challenge and you won't feel lethargic or exhausted.

After this, move towards a 10-hour eating window and slowly progress towards an 8-hour feeding window. This is the way to slowly teach your body how to deal with the changes induced by limited calorie intake.

Eating heavy meals after fasting. After fasting, when you are feeling hungry, it is normal to overeat, because your body was hungry.

But overeating and overloading on calories will kill the soul of fasting. This will flush down your entire day's effort and you won't be able to reap the benefits of fasting.

Especially when you are trying to lose weight, if you take much more calories than you lost during the fast, then you won't lose any weight.

Because the number of calories you gained due to overeating exceeded the number of calories you lost during your fast. A simple equation must be remembered for successful weight loss and that is the number of calories lost should be greater than the number of calories gained.

Also, if you are following shorter fasting periods and lose fewer calories, but then balance them out after eating, that won't also help you lose weight which will in return create an impression in your mind that Intermittent Fasting doesn't work.

Although, the blame for not losing weight goes on your extremely high-calorie intake after fast, yet you still end up quitting the healthy lifestyle of Intermittent Fasting.

An easy solution to this problem is that when you sit down to eat after your fast, do not pile up your plate with food. Instead, divide your food intake into several meals. A meal divided into several small portions is better than one huge meal.

Another mistake people make is to eat fast when hungry. When you eat fast, you end up eating more than needed. Eating slowly will help you satisfy your appetite by eating less.

It will give you a feeling of stomach-full after eating less. So, when you are trying to lose weight fast, avoid these eating mistakes and you will see the best results in no time.

Eating unhealthy. Some people think that Intermittent Fasting is a magical technique that will resolve all their problems on its own.

Yes, Intermittent Fasting is indeed an incredibly effective tool that will not help you to lose weight but will also restore your health.

Intermittent Fasting cannot work if you are consuming a diet full of processed foods and sugars so, when you are fasting, it becomes more important to nourish your body with healthy foods than before. During Intermittent Fasting, your body becomes much more dependent on the foods you eat.

So, Intermittent Fasting will work best if you eat healthy foods and won't work at all if you eat unhealthy foods. Intermittent Fasting is not just about the number of calories you consume, it's more about eating nutrient-dense foods.

Suppose you consume 500 calories of fruit one day and the next day you consume 500 calories of fried potato chips.

The day you had 500 healthy calories gained from eating fruit, that day you will observe higher energy levels, and overall healthy feeling, and higher stamina.

In contrast, when you had 500 calories of fried foods, it will not only keep your body from receiving nourishment but will also make it harder for you to fast. Try and maintain a balance of all macronutrients like iron, fiber, healthy fats, and carbs.

Your body needs all the possible nutrition since it is working hard to burn the excess fats from the body. So, don't make the rookie mistake of eating unhealthy foods and then claiming that Intermittent Fasting doesn't work.

It works best when you incorporate healthy and nutritious foods in your diet and keep a healthy schedule of fasting and eating.

Not drinking enough water/fluids. This is the most disastrous mistake anyone can make during Intermittent Fasting.

When your body is in a fast state, it starts to decompose the damaged components and detoxifies the body.

It is extremely important to flush out those toxins from your body by drinking plenty of water and other fluids. Ideally, you should drink more when you are fasting.

The absence of water won't allow the toxins to leave the body and thus will hurt your body rather than healing it.

During a fast, you miss out on the hydration that fruits and vegetables provide your body. Not drinking enough water will push your body into a state of dehydration. And you must note that dehydration leads to several hundred other problems like headaches, muscle cramps, and many others.

Sometimes you might feel intense hunger pangs during your fast and you might mistake them for happening because you are hungry. Sometimes, these pangs are a sign that your body is in dire need of water.

So, make sure to drink plenty of water during fasting, this will keep your body satiated during fasted windows. Plus, you will avoid many health problems caused by dehydration.

Forcing your body. Intermittent Fasting might not be the best option for every single human being. Each body is designed differently and it is quite possible that Intermittent Fasting doesn't work for you.

It has been reported several times that some people complain that they didn't lose any weight even after months and months of struggle and it is ok to acknowledge it.

Everything doesn't suit everyone. You do not need to go out of the way to force your body. Not each body is built for Intermittent Fasting.

If you are a woman that has a body type that carries extra fat all the time, then your metabolism may be slow.

Slow metabolism leads to late food digestion and this might not give enough time to your body to start burning fat during the fasted state. On the opposite, if you are a woman with a very fast metabolism and digestion, then you might find fasting extremely difficult to implement.

It is totally fine to listen to what your body is telling you and if it is telling you to stop and get it out of the misery then do so.

You do not need to force and push your body to must follow Intermittent Fasting. Forcing your body might produce even worse results and might perpetuate imbalance in your body.

If Intermittent Fasting feels like a continuous struggle and you are not getting used to the fasting schedules, then you do not need to drain your mental health. Just take a step back, re-evaluate the best method for you to opt for weight-loss.

Choosing the wrong Intermittent Fasting strategy. The biggest reason why any diet fails is because of their extreme contrast without daily life habits.

The intense schedules and strict calorie restrictions contrast hugely from their normal eating routine and that's why people often feel impossible to maintain such hardcore schedules.

Similarly, talking about Intermittent Fasting, if you are used to eating after every hour or two, then adapting alternate day fasting or an 8-hour eating window might feel impossible to you.

Sometimes you may rush into this and choose the wrong fasting style. If you don't have the potential of staying hungry then you should start from 12 or 14 hours of eating windows and slowly progress towards the 8-hours feeding window method.

Another easy way is to start with the 12/12 method. This will allow you a 12-hour fasting window and a 12-hour eating window.

You can further divide every 12 hours into a 6-6 hour strategy and this won't make you feel you are stepping into something extraordinarily tough. You have to work on fasting styles yourself and see what fits best for you.

But choosing the wrong method of fasting and then giving up on the entire practice is not a wise thing to do. Don't set yourself up for misery by signing up for something you already know is going to hinder your lifestyle.

Everyone has a different nature and attitude towards eating schedules. If you are used to staying awake at night, then don't plan to start your fast at 6 or 7 PM.

If you love to go to the gym every day, then don't choose a fasting plan that restricts your calorie consumption to a few days a week.

It is all dependent on you and your lifestyle; choose a fasting plan that you think you can do and can along with your lifestyle.

Take-away. YES, you might make some of these mistakes along the way during Intermittent Fasting. But it doesn't mean that you should give up on the entire method and claim that you cannot lose weight through Intermittent Fasting.

Each body is designed differently, so instead of rushing towards the decision that Intermittent Fasting doesn't work for you, perform some experiments with Intermittent Fasting methods and you never know the next method you try may suit your body completely and you successfully lose the extra weight.

It is not a hit-and-try method; in fact, it is the try-try again till you succeed method. If you started with weekly Intermittent Fasting and even after months you cannot see a significant change then it means that you made a mistake in judgment.

Your body is not facing a challenge in weekly fasting. You should up your game and go for daily fasting. All of this is dependent on your intuition and judgment. Making mistakes is fine, not learning from them is bad.

Precautionary measures for Intermittent Fasting

Overly restricting your calorie intake is not necessary. If you are in your initial days of Intermittent Fasting, you should start to slowly restrict your calorie intake so that your body can get used to less intake with time.

But if you have been practicing Intermittent Fasting for a long time now and you can easily pull-off an 8-hour feeding window method or daily Intermittent Fasting, then you don't need to worry about your calorie intake.

The reason is that your body is going through a long fasting window and providing necessary nutrition is important. Keeping track of calorie intake and overly obsessing about it is unnecessary.

The key is to be consistent with the feeding and fasting schedules and if you are regularly following the schedule then calorie intake should be the least of your worries.

Do keep a general track and balance of the foods you consume, meaning if you had junk food for one meal then do balance it out with a healthy meal afterward.

Making your meal portion smaller with time is a good practice for Intermittent Fasting and can help you in many ways. But over-doing can create deficiencies in your body. If you feel like you are hungry even after a small meal then enjoying a healthy snack afterward can never hurt you.

It's just that your body is telling you it needs more food and it is common to feel after a long fast. Thus, don't overly restrict your calorie intake, there is no hard and fast rule on the calorie intake in Intermittent Fasting and it's healthy to keep it that way.

Don't overdo it or go over-board. Some people are more eager than others to lose weight and integrate different Intermittent Fasting methods for a better and faster result.

Because of their eagerness, they might go over-board with fasting and it can turn out to be too much for their bodies. Women are already sensitive to the levels of insulin and if a slow and regular approach is not adopted, they might end up exhausting themselves too fast.

If you started with a 12-hour window of eating and fasting, then you might feel pretty confident about the fact that you can easily fast without any problem for longer durations.

After that, if you directly jump to an 8-hour feeding window, it might extremely difficult for you to manage the hunger levels.

A 12-hour window is not very different from your normal routine, so keep in mind that progressing consistently though slowly is more beneficial rather than getting excited and putting your body through too much and end up going over-board.

This will exhaust you faster and you will lose interest in the entire method just because of over-doing it.

Beware of what fluids to consume during the 'fasting window'. As discussed earlier, many fluids and beverages out there in the market wearing a label of sugar-free are not sugar-free at all.

They do add some artificial flavors or sweeteners instead of sugar to make it taste good. Beware of such drinks! They can take you right out of the fasting cycle and can also spike up your insulin and sugar levels in the body.

Always go for water, sparkling or mineral or lime. You can also drink black coffee and various types of unsweetened tea.

Consumption of fluids is although very important during fasting intervals but you have to be cautious about the nature of the drinks. A sugary drink will leave you with an instant sugar-high and then during your fast when your insulin level drops, you will suddenly crave those sugary drinks.

This makes it much harder for a person to fast for longer periods. Keeping your body hydrated during the fasting window carries vital significance for the health of your body.

If you keep following the fast and feeding window properly and manage to fast for longer periods but forget to keep your fluid intake high; then your entire struggle can go down the drain.

Intermittent Fasting burns your fat and decomposes it into toxins, and to get rid of those harmful toxins, you need to flush them out by drinking lots and lots of fluids.

Never underestimate the power of drinking water during a fast. It will keep you satiated during the fast as well as it will get rid of the harmful side-effects of dehydration.

Focus on 'when' rather than 'what'. Intermittent Fasting emphasizes eating schedule meaning 'when' and does not give much focus on 'what' to eat.

Eating schedules, fasting, and feeding windows carry more importance than what foods to eat to eat after fasting. If you focus on what to eat then you might neglect the importance of following fasting schedules.

A balanced diet is although important in Intermittent Fasting but when you are talking about losing weight, calorie intake doesn't matter much. What matters is that you fast and enable your body to enter into the fat-burning mode.

To lose weight, it is obvious that you have to get rid of the existing fat inside your body.

And to that, your body needs to learn that when your insulin levels are low, that is you are under a fasting state, the body needs to burn existing fat present inside your fat cells.

This helps the process of calorie burning and thus acts as a pioneer for weight-loss.

Therefore, as a precautionary measure, stop worrying and fussing about calorie intake, what foods to avoid, and foods to eat and solely focus on your fasting windows. The longer the fasting window, the higher the fat burn, more the weight-loss.

Don't be hesitant in 'eating enough' during your feeding window. Eating enough and over-eating are two very different things. Eating enough means enjoying an amount of meal that sufficiently satiates your hunger and satisfies your appetite. Over-eating means to eat more than the demand of your body.

Intermittent Fasting doesn't place any bounds on what foods to eat, but just like any other weight-loss program, over-eating doesn't prove beneficial here as well.

On the other hand, eating less than your appetite might also not prove healthy for some people. When you are not feeling full and want to eat more, it means that your body needs more nutrition.

And to maintain a healthy body and a healthy lifestyle, you need to fulfill the nutrition requirements of your body. So never feel hesitant in satisfying your appetite. Eat enough but don't over-eat.

Female hormonal balance and Intermittent Fasting

Intermittent Fasting affects women differently than men and there are several plausible reasons for it. Women have high sensitivity to hormonal changes.

Female bodies trigger hunger hormones faster than a man's body when under the state called fasted state or underfed state.

Women need to know that their bodies are not as much tougher as men's bodies, and they should treat their bodies accordingly.

It is possible that a male member of your family is practicing a 24-hour Intermittent Fasting schedule and does not feel even a little weak or low on energy.

But if you try this schedule, it gets too much for you. This is normal and there is nothing to worry about here. Many hormones inside a woman's body get triggered way faster than men's.

That's why there are more considerations for women than men related to Intermittent Fasting.

There are a few factors that induce hormonal imbalance in women and those are:

- Extreme stress (physical or mental)
- Not enough sleep
- Exercising way too much
- Not eating enough
- Not eating healthy

These are some of the reasons why your body might be under a hormonal imbalance. Intermittent Fasting is known to improve metabolic rates and restore hormonal balance.

If you follow Intermittent Fasting correctly and avoid the above-mentioned conditions, you will not only lose weight but you will also heal and nourish your body.

Intermittent Fasting allows you to start slow, don't 'shock' your hormones by extreme starvation, and maintain a healthy eating pattern.

Regular eating intervals and a healthier diet will help your body to fight with such imbalances. And Intermittent Fasting offers the best eating patterns to its practitioners.

How does IF affect women differently than men?

Women tend to implement various ways for fast weight loss like exercising, workouts, different kinds of dieting, etc. All the above-mentioned ways are artificial weight loss techniques because you are not losing weight naturally.

You are putting your body through a lot of pressure to shed-off the extra pounds. Intermittent Fasting has proven the most effective and beneficial technique for women.

It takes a natural way to lose weight and does not create any nutrition deficiencies. Women need higher nutrition than men and are more sensitive to signs of starvation. They need all sorts of vitamins and minerals to keep a healthy body.

They have the responsibility of managing the entire household, take care of their family, juggle work, and also give birth to a new person.

So, strict dieting and cutting-off nutrition can seriously harm the health of a woman. It might induce hormonal imbalance, hundreds of deficiencies, and weaknesses.

Therefore, IF brings a safe and easy way for all the women out there to safely achieve their goal weight without stressing their bodies and without removing necessary nutrients from their life.

Note! Extreme calorie restriction can hinder female hormones and can cause problems like hormonal imbalance, infertility, and irregular periods.

This is why women who are intermittently fasting mustn't be doing it to restrict their calorie intake, they should opt for this for better health and wellness aspects.

The reason is that when extreme restrictions are induced on calorie intake, it slows down the metabolism and hinders the digestive system.

It might make your digestive system slow too and this will put your hormones out of balance and won't allow your body to function at the most optimal levels.

Ask yourself and your body, Extreme or Moderate? This means that if your body tells you that you are pushing it way too much or forcing it too much then it means you are on extreme levels of calorie restriction.

And if your body feels well and fine during a fast because you eat healthy afterward, it means that it's under a moderate state of calorie intake. Intermittent Fasting boosts energy levels, increases stamina, increases motivation and it also improves cognitive functions.

Women need higher energy levels and strict dieting will drastically decrease these levels. A slow and steady approach to limit the food intake is the best and safest approach here.

Intermittent Fasting defines specific eating windows and complements a healthy diet and lifestyle.

Chapter 4

When should women avoid Intermittent Fasting?

There are times when women should avoid any diet plans or even Intermittent Fasting. This includes:

- Pregnancy
- Nursing
- Under chronic stress
- Having a history of eating disorders
- Having an irregular sleep pattern

How IF helps women? Women's bodies are designed in such a way that it maintains prime fertility conditions so that they don't have to face fertility problems later. And this is the main reason why female hormones are much active and more sensitive than male hormones.

It has been revealed through studies that starvation and stress when mix together, can negatively affect the fertility of a woman.

This means that if a woman is following extreme dieting plans and long starvation hours plus she is facing constant stress, then she may be hurting her health.

Intermittent Fasting is advantageous for women in this regard because unlike diets, women can choose however long they want to fast, depending upon their stamina and energy.

If you are a working woman and several days of the week you work too hard or remain under stress, then you can easily opt not to fast on those days.

Just simply choose the days of the week in which you have low work pressure and lower stress. You can do this through a "weekly Intermittent Fasting" schedule and just choose 2 days of the week that you can easily carry a fast.

Unlike diet programs; Intermittent Fasting cares about your health; both mental and physical. Intermittent Fasting creates a healthy eating schedule that simplifies your life thus reducing mental pressure. It also makes you follow a healthy diet plan which helps you to stay more active and productive.

This increases your physical health. Diets will leave your body all lazy and weak and they can also trigger hormonal imbalance.

Pros and cons of IF for women

Must Note! Cons can only occur if you overly restrict your calorie intake, eat unhealthily, go past the limits of fasting windows, and fast more than 24 hours.

Pros	Cons
Sustainable weight loss	Disturbed metabolism
Increase in muscle mass	Irregular periods
Higher energy levels	Fertility issues
Reduction in inflammation	Anxiety
Improved insulin sensitivity	Difficulty in sleeping
Reduced oxidative stress	Shrinking of ovaries
Boosts up cognitive functions	Hormonal imbalance

7-Day Intermittent Fasting Guide for Beginners

To help you kick-start your Intermittent Fasting journey, here is a simple and easy to follow 7-Day guide. If you have never tried Intermittent Fasting before and you are just starting your journey, then here is a convenient 7-day plan laid out for you so that you have a fun, easy, and good experience.

The tasks and the goals for each day are specifically provided so that you don't start too rash or make any mistake. For your first week, you should slowly ease into Intermittent Fasting so that your body doesn't go into a shocking state.

DAY 1:

Fasting Window	Feeding window
12 hours	12 hours

For the very first day of the first week, you should start by choosing a convenient fasting and feeding window. This 12-hour window is not very different from your daily life and it will not pressurize your body on the very first day.

The main goal of this activity and beginner's guide is to highlight the fact that you should slowly ease into the journey of Intermittent Fasting.

If you start hard and don't give enough time to your body to adjust, then chances are that you will torment your health and might put your hormones into a shocked state.

Going too fast too soon can create many imbalances like hormonal imbalance or metabolite imbalance.

12-hour fasting and 12-hour feeding window mean that you only have to fast for half a day. In our normal routine, the gaps between our meals add up to almost 12 hours and this doesn't differentiate much from our normal routine.

Thus, this makes it easier for your brain and body to get used to and prepare for some eating changes. It will also give you more time to settle in and adjust to the new fasting schedules.

Intermittent Fasting though offers different kinds of programs for different people, but this guide will eventually put you with the **8-hour feeding window method.** That is, on Day 7, you will be starting with the 8-hour feeding and 16-hour fasting window method. And you will continue with the most on the following days.

Once you feel comfortable with this method, you can further shorten your feeding window and elongate your fasting cycle. It all depends on your body, if it allows you to stretch the cycles you can.

And if not, then keep following an 8-hour method and with the time you will see the results that you have been looking for.

The Goal of Day 1: For your day 1, you only have to choose your Intermittent Fasting schedule. Today's goal is very easy and very doable for you. You have to see, which fasting schedule best suits your lifestyle and routine and the schedule you want to follow after your initial training.

The best thing is that for your first 7 days, you explore all fasting options while simultaneously putting your body in a habit of fasting slowly and steadily.

After the 7 days complete, you can choose any Intermittent Fasting schedule; weekly, daily, or even alternate fasting schedules. Stay consistent and keep following the 7-day guide and this will prove to be the most contributing factor to your success.

DAY 2:

Fasting Window	Feeding window
13 hours	11 hours

On day 2, your fasting window is extended to 13 hours. Just one hour more than yesterday. You can do it!

Gradually increasing the window will allow your body to understand the new changes and will allow it to handle the new calorie intake. If you are suddenly start-off with alternate-day fasting which has a 2-hour feeding and fasting cycle, then your body will get confused on how to deal with such a big change in such a short time.

Now, you are getting familiar with how Intermittent Fasting works. It might be possible that you don't feel much different than before which is a good sign. It means that your body is comfortable with the new fasting cycles. And if you are already feeling some low energy levels then there is nothing to worry about!

Usually, all bodies take a 7 or 10 day time to adjust to this fasting schedule. That is why this guide is introduced so that you don't get afraid or anxious and quit Intermittent Fasting without giving it a worthy shot.

Day 2 will introduce you to new healthy guidelines that support your goals of Intermittent Fasting. Guidelines will help you in losing weight and can also assist you in maintaining a healthier lifestyle.

Define your fasting goals and what you want to achieve by the end of the day. Either your goal is to just lose weight or if your goal is to learn and apply healthy eating schedules; simply focus on eating healthy and avoid the stress of counting calories.

Eat until you satisfy your appetite and remember not to overeat! Intermittent Fasting cannot work until your body knows how to burn the fat inside the body. So, for that purpose, do not overeat. Eat just enough to satiate your appetite.

The Goal of Day 2: Today's goal is to learn the basics of Intermittent Fasting. Learn about the importance of eating whole foods and avoiding processed foods and sugar.

Learn about healthy carbs and empty carbs. Get to know about the significance of eating all types of healthy foods and provide all necessary nutrition to your body during the feeding window.

Think about what simple yet delicious meals you can prepare for yourself at home.

Familiarize yourself with healthy fluids like water, black coffee, and tea.

Avoid sugary drinks like juices, sodas, and diet sodas. Learn about the benefits and advantages of keeping yourself hydrated during your fast and also get to know what happens if you let your body dehydrate.

Several hundred problems are born if you don't keep yourself hydrated, so make sure to drink plenty of fluids!

DAY 3:

Fasting Window	Feeding window
14 hours	10 hours

Day 3 is here with an increase of one more hour in the fasting window. Do not worry at all because you are capable of doing this!

This guide is specially designed for beginners and it won't affect your health until you keep enjoying healthy meals.

You are moving gradually and consistently and you should appreciate yourself for it. Each day, your body is getting stronger and stronger.

With each day passing, you are adapting to a healthier lifestyle and better eating patterns.

Stay active and be productive. Don't let the concept fool you that since you are fasting you should reduce your activities and rest more. This won't help you. You have to get your body used to the fact that you will work just like you used to, the difference is that you are limiting your food intake to specific hours of the day.

Eating at better times will give you more energy to carry out your tasks of the day. Again, you might have some concerns if you are feeling tired and low on energy. Don't worry as there is nothing unusual going on. It is normal to feel a bit tired at the beginning of this journey and you have to give 4 to 6 more days to your body if you want to decide that either you want to continue or not.

Don't think of giving up earlier than 10 days. It usually takes 7 to 10 days for a human body to adjust to fasting. Believe that you can do it and know that you are not the first one fasting.

Humans have been fasting for thousands of years now and their bodies are well capable of it. If they can, so can you! Just remain consistent.

The Goal of Day 3: Today's goal is to define your reward! Defining your reward will keep you enthused and will inspire you to keep the hard work up. You can define a reward for each day that you successfully fast or you can define a big reward when the 7 days end.

The reward can be a simple cheering sentence like "Good job! You are doing great! Yes, you can do this!" or can be a bigger reward than this like a day out or a treat to go to a restaurant.

Small rewards help you keep your spirits high and you remind yourself of what you can achieve. Saying these small sentences will help you to keep continuing until you achieve your goal weight.

Bigger rewards are for people who find fasting difficult, they want to lose weight but they don't want to limit their eating habits.

For such purpose, you can promise yourself something like 'if you lose a pound a week, you will get to treat yourself at a restaurant after that week'.

These are just ways and tricks to keep yourself continue on the journey of Intermittent Fasting and one day reach your goal of weight or a healthier lifestyle.

DAY 4:

Fasting Window	Feeding window
15 hours	9 hours

Congratulations! You are more than halfway there.

Today, you will be fasting for 15 hours already. The beauty of this technique is that it doesn't let you feel way out of routine and yet you are significantly progressing towards your goal each day.

You might already be seeing the healthy effects of an Intermittent Fasting schedule. You might feel you already have lost a little bit of weight but it is also normal not to feel a change just about now.

Be patient! Each body is designed differently and everyone has a different metabolism rate. You don't need to worry if you have a slow or fast metabolism; just keep going on with this fasting schedule and your goal will not appear far away from you.

If you are feeling extreme hunger pangs during your fast, it might be a signal that you are not eating healthy enough or you are drinking fewer fluids than needed. Remember; do not dehydrate yourself during your fast.

Also, beware of avoiding sugary fluids during your fast. Sugary fluids can break your fast and throw you out of the fasting cycle.

We want a healthier body, not an even weaker body than before. And to deal with the problem of not eating enough healthy foods, today's goal is to have a very healthy meal rich in protein and nutrition.

The Goal of Day 4: Today's goal is to prepare a high protein meal. Eating healthy and fulfilling your nutrition needs is necessary for success in Intermittent Fasting. So, today you are going to make yourself a protein-filled lunch.

The protein can be of your choice like fish, grilled meat, eggs, beans, or tofu. You can pair it up with steamed or grilled veggies and you will have a nutrition-dense meal in front of you.

Women need all the possible nutrition during the feeding cycle.

So, to keep yourself healthy and active, and to avoid nutrition problems, enjoy a healthy meal daily. Intermittent Fasting doesn't restrict you on calorie intake.

It also doesn't restrict you on what foods to eat. But eating healthy at least once a day during fasting days is very important in maintaining a good and healthy body.

DAY 5:

Fasting Window	Feeding window
16 hours	8 hours

You have successfully reached the 16/8 window goal. You will today be fasting for 16 hours with an 8-hour feeding window.

Since you have been progressing slowly, today you won't feel it very hard to fast for 16 hours. But if you had started directly from a 16-hour schedule, you would have been feeling very tired, exhausted, and lazy.

Following this guide has helped you to successfully reach your goal of fasting without putting your body through drastic changes.

Research has shown that hundreds of people have undertaken similar challenges. Some people have taken a 21-day fasting challenge and some went for a shorter challenge.

But the results for all such challenges have been positive and satisfying.

These types of challenges also highlight the significance of taking it slow but they also challenge your body a little bit.

Some people are satisfied with the results of these challenges while some are left behind because they have a slower pace than others and cannot keep up with the challenge.

This 7-day guide is designed for all kinds of people. If you had no problem until now; then very well! Keep it up!

But if you anytime feel that this is too much for your body then you can pause at whatever day you are and practice it for a few more days.

For example, if you are on day 3 where you have a 14/10 window ratio and you felt that it was a little hard for you and you need more time to adjust, then there is nothing to worry about.

Make day 4 also a 14/10 window and keep going until you are comfortable with it and then move on.

The Goal of day 5: The goal for day 5 is to drink fluids like green tea or black coffee if you feel hungry. This will help you go through with 16 hours fast easily and will also curb your hunger. Also, keep in mind that water is the best fluid to drink during the fast.

But if you want to curb your hunger a little bit you can drink these green tea or black coffee too. But don't overdo it! Black coffee is rich in antioxidants and also greatly helps to suppress hunger.

But you have to remember that you cannot add milk, cream, or sugar to your coffee. This will increase your sugar and insulin levels and thus will be counted as eating.

Similarly, if you want to drink tea instead of coffee, it is better to have green tea and it must be unsweetened. Sugar is a no-no in any case during your fast. So, sugar in any form should be avoided because it can instigate hunger.

DAY 6:

Fasting Window	Feeding window
16 hours	8 hours

Today you are staying with yesterday's schedule that is 16 hours fast and an 8-hour feeding window. This right here is an Intermittent Fasting method and you do not need to go further if you don't want to.

This is called the 8-hour feeding window method and you can stick to it if you are comfortable with how things are right now.

If you are looking for a harder challenge then you should practice two more days; day 6 and day 7 with the same schedule and then move forward to something hard.

Practicing the schedule, a little more will help you build your stamina for a much harder challenge and you will not face any difficulty once you move past this level. Just keep on going as you are, follow the schedule, keep eating healthy, and be consistent no matter what!

Don't get overconfident and be too quick about it. If you didn't have any problem until now, it's good. But it doesn't mean that you are ready for anything to be put in front of you.

Do not mess up everything by going too fast. You are in a great condition right now; follow this schedule for two more days and then move on to your decided Intermittent Fasting schedule.

It is totally good and fine to stay here and practice as long as you want. Get used to it, no matter how much time it takes.

The Goal for Day 6: The goal for the day is to go for a walk. If you already walk daily or you are already used to exercising a little bit daily, then it's great! Your job for the day is done. But if you haven't stayed much active during these fasting days, then start today.

It's your second day following the 16/8 schedule, so don't worry about exhausting yourself. Your body knows that it has an 8-hour feeding window allowed and it will function optimally.

Walking will also switch your focus from hunger and will help you pass the last hours of fasting much more conveniently. There is just a slight need of staying active and increasing daily activity.

The purpose is to build stamina in your body for physical activities during Intermittent Fasting.

So, start with a small walk if you are not in a habit of it or walk as much you like if your body allows you.

Remember to listen to your body. When you feel tired, stop, and go home. Tomorrow you will have much higher stamina and you will probably walk double than today.

DAY 7:

Fasting Window	Feeding window
16 hours	8 hours

Today you keep your new 16/8 fasting schedule. While doing so, you will do some reflection on how your past week went.

You will answer some common survey questions that people usually take at the end of this process. These questions will help you assess the overall experience.

After you answer these questions to yourself, you will decide whether you want to continue with this schedule, or do you want to shift to some other fasting schedule?

The questions are as follows:

- How do you feel during and after your fast?
- Do you feel tired or fatigued?
- Is there any change in your energy levels?
- How was the experience? Did you enjoy it or was it torture for you?
- Have you noticed any change in your overall mood?
- How is your skin's condition? Is it better than before or does it feel dry?
- What was your biggest struggle?
- Is there any change that you would like to implement?
- Does this schedule suit your lifestyle?

The Goal of Day 7: Today your goal is to decide which schedule of Intermittent Fasting to follow? You will answer the above-mentioned questions and that will help you decide if you want to stick with the existing schedule or do you want a bigger challenge?

You will assess how well your last week went and was it even a challenge for you or not? If it didn't feel like much of a challenge then go for even shorter feeding cycles.

But if it was too much to take then either elongate the feeding window or move towards a weekly fasting schedule. Feel free to say out loud whatever you are thinking. There is nothing to be ashamed of.

Thousands of people decide that this is too much and they need to go towards a lighter fasting schedule. They go for what their body tells them and after a year or so they happily report back with the great news that they achieved their goal weight and that they are very happy now.

Thus, follow your gut, openly answer the questions, and strategize your plan. This will help you accelerate the decision-making process and you will be able to make Intermittent Fasting a new sustainable habit.

Is Exercise Safe for women during IF?

It all depends upon your stamina. Generally, women who exercise during Intermittent Fasting have had no problems.

They report that it keeps them active and helps to burn more fat and thus weight loss is pretty fast. Exercise can greatly help with fat-adaptation.

Glycogen (the stored form of glucose in your liver and muscles that helps the body when you are under a fast) gets depleted when you fast or sleep and further depletes when you exercise.

What's the benefit of this? This will increase insulin sensitivity.

That means that when you have a meal after a workout, it will be much efficiently utilized by the body since it kept burning fat during the entire time.

A meal after a workout will be stored in the form of glycogen in muscles while some of it is utilized to get the energy of the body back up. The least amounts are stored as fats and it can prove extremely beneficial for you when your goal is to lose weight.

Our body follows a simple rule of "Higher insulin levels, higher fat storage" and vice versa. Therefore, keeping insulin levels low is very important when you are trying to lose weight and exercise is one of the best ways to do it.

When insulin sensitivity is at a normal level, the food consumed will be utilized for full glycogen storage in muscles; it will also be used as glucose in the bloodstream and thus has a higher chance to get stored in the form of fat.

A good workout can help you regulate and increase your insulin sensitivity.

How to lower insulin levels (How to increase insulin sensitivity)? Few things can help to increase insulin sensitivity and those are:

- Intermittent Fasting
- Exercise
- Low carb diet
- Low-calorie diet
- Nutrient-dense foods

Safety concerns about exercising during fasting: Although it sounds like exercise is the best and fastest option to lose weight. But some precautions need to be considered before jumping to a decision.

Long fasts and long workouts might push your body to start breaking down the muscle to use protein as fuel.

This can hurt your lean muscle mass. Women who like to have abdominal muscles or arm muscles should note that extreme deprivation from food and extreme hard workouts will eventually take a toll on your muscle mass.

So, if you want to maintain your muscle mass but want to lose weight, then do exercise but remain at a moderate level of exercising. Don't work out too hard and for too much longer durations.

How to safely exercise while fasting? If your ultimate goal is to reduce body fat while maintaining your fitness level and muscle mass then you need to keep your body in the safe zone. Listed below are some tips to successfully achieve your goal while exercising:

1) **The duration and intensity should be low**
   When a longer duration of exercising is paired up with long fasts, your body can enter into a state of calorie deficiency. And to refuel itself, it will start to burn protein and energy present in the muscles. If you push yourself too hard, you can end up feeling dizzy or even light-headed. When this happens, relax and take a step back. Because it is a clear sign that you are forcing your body too much. Keep the intensity of the workout low too. Extremely hard workouts can create energy deficiency in your body. Therefore, just keep the duration and intensity of the exercise at a low level.
2) **Stay hydrated and keep your electrolytes up**
   During fasting, you should increase your water intake no matter if you exercise or not. Dehydration can cause several problems like headaches and it can also slow down the metabolism. If you are exercising as well as fasting, make sure to focus on keeping yourself hydrated and keeping your electrolytes up. Choose a good low-calorie hydration source and stick with it throughout the process. Avoid sports drinks because they are extremely high in sugar and your goal is to lower the insulin levels, not spike them up.
3) **Eat a meal closer to your workout**
   It is a misconception that you should not eat close to your workout session. Always prefer eating a meal after a workout because that will help your body to get the most out of the food. Having a meal shortly after exercise will help your muscles to regain strength because it will provide glycogen to them. The chances of food getting stored as fat

become very low because your body balances out its fuel needs and utilizes them properly.

4) **Listen to your body**

   The most important thing is to listen to your body. If you are feeling dizzy or light-headed then you may be having very low blood sugar levels. It is also a sign of dehydration. So, in such a case, go for a healthy drink and then have a nutritious and well-balanced meal. After that, reanalyze your workout style. It might be possible that you are pushing your body way too hard and you need to take a step back and shift towards a relatively low-intensity exercise.

Conclusion: Exercise does not suit everyone while fasting. It may or may not work out for you. Some people feel perfectly healthy and more active when they indulge in a light exercise with a fast while others may not feel comfortable with exercise at all.

If your workouts are getting weaker as a result of fasting; it might be a sign that your body needs more nutrition or you need to try some other Intermittent Fasting schedule. And if the rest of your fasting cycle is working great for you but when you exercise you feel exhausted, then you need to ease up on exercising or workout methods.

Remember, always move steadily and start with low intensity; either it is exercise or it is Intermittent Fasting. Knowing when to back-off is important when you are trying both Intermittent Fasting as well as exercising.

Chapter 5

Why is Autophagy important for women?

What is Autophagy? Autophagy is a process in which the body cleans out the damaged cells and then generates new and healthier cells. It is like a self-preservation system through which the body itself locates and removes the dysfunctional cells or repairs them.

Even healthy human bodies experience cell damaging. As a result of our metabolic processes, it is very natural that cells constantly become damaged. Sometimes, with increased stress, the damaged cells also radically increase. And that's why nature introduced autophagy in our bodies.

Autophagy helps the body to clear out damaged cells or cells that have no functional purpose in the body. Such non-functional cells keep lingering inside our bodies until they are cleared out. Clearing them out is very important because if such damaged cells don't clear out from our bodies, we can become more susceptible to diseases and illnesses.

Is autophagy good for health? Researchers have proven that autophagy acts as a survival mechanism for our bodies and it's a way for the body to protect itself. Studies have also shown that autophagy is important in "cleaning up of the body" and acts as a defense strategy against higher stress levels. So yes, it is good for our bodies. It is key in preventing various types of diseases like cancer, liver disease, diabetes, autoimmune diseases, and infections.

The relation between autophagy and Intermittent Fasting: To induce autophagy, Intermittent Fasting plays a significantly important role. To say that Intermittent Fasting causes the autophagy process to start won't be wrong. Different schedules of Intermittent Fasting can induce autophagy in a body including daily Intermittent Fasting (with a few hours of eating window) or alternate Intermittent Fasting (where you fast for 24 hours and then can eat for the next 24 hours).

Another easier way to induce autophagy through Intermittent Fasting is to eat one or two meals a day with a solid gap between them and don't snack in between. Staying hungry between several intervals will initiate low insulin levels inside your body and that acts as a signal that now the body needs fuel and it can only get from inside a body. That's when it starts burning fat as well as clears out hazardous and damaged cells. That's how Intermittent Fasting plays a role in healing and restoring health to a body.

Benefits of Autophagy:

- Unnecessary and dysfunctional cells are disassembled and cleared out from the body.
- It helps to fight infectious diseases.
- It strengthens the immune system.
- Prevents cancer and various other neurodegenerative diseases.
- Provides the cells with molecular energy.
- Recycles damaged proteins and regulates the functions of the cells.
- Protects the nervous system.
- Enhances the growth of the brain and nerve cells.
- Improves the strength and cognitive functions of the brain.
- Protects against heart diseases and helps in the growth of heart cells.
- Provides stability of DNA
- Prevents any damage to healthy organs and body tissues
- The mechanism that has anti-aging benefits.

Importance of autophagy for women: It is quite normal for women to have a hormonal imbalance. Sometimes it happens because of disturbed metabolism and sometimes you may never know the reason. In case when you don't know the reason for the imbalance, autophagy can come in and greatly help you. It restores the balance of your hormonal cells and can also discard any harmful or dysfunctional cells. Thus, for restoring your hormonal imbalance or for the regulation of disorders; autophagy can play an important role.

And to induce autophagy you need to intermittently fast.

Secondly, Breast cancer is the most common and fatal cancer in women worldwide. A study has shown that roughly over a million women are diagnosed with breast cancer in a year. Though with the advancement of the medical field it is not considered fatal now.

Cancer development can be controlled through autophagy. It hinders the way of progression of cancer and removes the growth of the defective cells. Autophagy plays a very important role in stopping the initiation of such canceled cells and if they have initiated already then autophagy stops their progression and discards those harmful cells out of our body. So, it is proved that autophagy is vastly beneficial for women. But again, the question stands:

How to initiate autophagy inside the body? Autophagy needs the triggering of cells and nothing triggers the cells better than Intermittent Fasting. So, fasting does not only help in losing weight, it also helps to induce autophagy inside a body which gets rids of all dysfunctional cells from the body. Thus, leaves your body healthier and fitter than before. Sometimes, health-care providers suggest Intermittent Fasting for overweight women because excess weight is making them susceptible to many diseases. The reason why the medical practitioner or the doctor might suggest Intermittent Fasting is because they want to strengthen your immune system to fight against diseases that might occur due to obesity. So, don't worry about the extra fat on your body, it can be easily gotten rid-off.

Start Intermittent Fasting with an easy to follow schedule, will not only help you with weight loss but will also help you increase health by inducing autophagy in your body. While Intermittent Fasting gets rid of your excess fat, autophagy will automatically get rid of dangerous and dysfunctional cells from your body.

Keys to improving general health

1) Be active. Staying active has numerous advantages for physical as well as mental health. Physical activity has hundreds of benefits and all of them can never be listed here. The most important benefit of staying active in the prevention of chronic diseases.

Researchers believe that staying physically active can prevent many illnesses and diseases while it also cures mental problems like anxiety, stress, and even depression. A healthy body just demands a little bit of daily exercise or walking or playing a game outside. It does not demand extreme hardcore workouts from you.

When it comes to physical health, there is a rule that the longer the better. It means if you walk for longer periods of stay physically active for a long time, then it helps to build higher stamina in your body. Physical movement can also help with weight-loss. It is because when your body is physically active and under motion, the body is constantly burning extra calories and fats for energy.

Staying active helps to build higher energy levels and lowers the fat levels. If you stay put and don't move around much, then the calories you daily consume have no way to burn themselves. As a result, they keep on piling up and you keep on gaining weight.

Therefore, stay physically active. It will solve almost all your health problems.

2) Have a healthy diet. People underestimate the power of a healthy diet. Because they are too busy with their lives, they don't have enough time to prepare a healthy and proper meal for themselves. Instead, they go ahead and eat whatever is available to them. Crappy foods will not be able to provide your body with any energy whatsoever. After eating, very soon you will feel you are hungry again and it's because they didn't have any nutritional value in them. If you have a busy work schedule, it is more of a reason to eat too healthy. Eating unhealthy can put the female hormonal balance into a state of chaos. Female bodies need a much more nutritious supply of food than men. It's because female bodies are designed to keep themselves running at optimal conditions so that they can go through childbirth and breastfeeding successfully. If your body doesn't receive nutrition enough for itself, how can it help you to have a healthy baby? Include everything in your meal including iron, protein, healthy fats, and carbs. Don't restrict yourself to low-carb diet plans because this won't allow your body to receive complete nutrition which it is supposed to. A healthy eating, healthy lifestyle!

3) Maintain a healthy body weight. Healthy body weight is defined by body mass index (BMI) and it ranges between 18 and 24 if you going for normal BMI. With the advancement of science, there have been many studies conducted and there are several ways to calculate your BMI. The easiest way to do it is from online BMI calculators. You can find many online BMI calculators that ask you your height and weight in lbs. and it tells you your BMI and it also tells you if it is healthy or not. If it is in a healthy range it will tell you that you have a normal BMI. If it is too high or too low, it will tell you that you have an unhealthy or abnormal BMI and you need to make efforts for a healthy and normal BMI.

Don't always focus on dieting and losing fats. Your body needs some energy sources, so better keep it that way. A few extra pounds won't hurt you until and unless you are maintaining a healthy diet. Although, if you are not eating healthy or at regular times, then your bodyweight gain may be a symbol of something else. For the body to work optimally, it needs proper nutrition, a healthy diet, and a well-maintained eating schedule. This allows you to stay from hundreds of problems like eating disorders, sleeping unwell, being more disposed to the diseases. Therefore, keep your focus on eating healthy and maintaining a healthy body weight.

4) Enjoy light exercise daily. Daily exercise has proven to be beneficial for the human body and numerous studies have been conducted for it. Results showed that women who exercise daily; not extreme hardcore workouts, just some light exercise showed better metabolic rates, higher digestion rate, and better ability to get rid of the excess fats. Staying active is always suggested by health-practitioners and doctors because it helps the immune system to grow stronger and helps it to fight off several diseases. It also helps to maintain a better physical as well as mental balance. If you are stressed out too much, go for a walk and it is guaranteed that it will calm your nerves by releasing toxins out of your body. Some women enjoy a healthy workout while some are not comfortable with exercising. Those who work out daily should remember not to overdo it overstretch it and keep the workout at a normal level. If you work out extremely hard daily then once you give it up, it will do more harm than good. And women who are not in a habit of daily physical exercise should start by taking baby steps. Go for a small walk today and gradually increase your walk time and pace. When you build up enough stamina, your body will itself tell you what to do next. Mobilization of stored fats is necessary when you are trying to lose weight. Just cutting off your diet supply might not do the magic. But throw in a light daily exercise; you will see your dream weight coming.

5) Think positive and stop stressing out. Research shows a healthy positive attitude helps in building a healthier and stronger immune system and boosts overall health. Your body will believe whatever you think, so think positively and focus on positive aspects of things in life and your body will also stay happy and positive. People with extremely busy work schedules and a hard lifestyle must do some positive thinking in a day; it will energize their bodies and keep them enthused. Stress is a very common mental disease observed in people these days. They don't eat healthily and keep stressing out, which plays a great hand in destroying the immune system, destroying the metabolic rate, increases the chances of heart problems, and dysfunctions in the digestive system. On top of that, it stresses out your brain and nerve cells and constantly keeps on making nerve cells damaged or even dysfunctional. Whenever you feel stressed, just stop for one moment, close your eyes and take a few deep breaths. Deep breaths help slow-down the heart rate.

People who have lower resting heart rates are usually in a better physical condition than those who have higher rates. You can also practice meditation and light exercise. Prolonged stress to the heart can induce many health problems like high blood pressure, depression, and obesity.

6) Shift to 5 small meals instead of 3 big ones. What, when, and how much you eat affects directly your metabolism and energy levels. Suppose that after a long day of hard work, you missed a meal and when you get home, you overeat because you feel so hungry. This overeating will affect you in so many ways that you can't even imagine. It will slow down your metabolism, it will make you feel lazy and lethargic and it will put your digestive system out of order.

Therefore, shift to a 5 meal schedule, where you enjoy 5 small meals in a day. This will save you from getting overweight, you will avoid cravings and it will help you to maintain your cool and balance. A smaller meal will eliminate the chances of overeating and thus helps you stay active. A huge meal will slow down your body and make you lazy, it is because your metabolism slows down and the body has to work hard to digest the meal. That's why you feel exhausted even after having a meal and you wonder why it is happening. Whenever you get a chance, divide your meals further. If you were going to have fried vegetables with a piece of grilled meat, then divide it into two portions and finish it in two meals. Or enjoy the meat now and then eat vegetables later. This will keep your metabolic rate up and you will feel energetic after eating and not lazy. It will also help your body to get the most out of a meal and not just store it up in the form of fats.

7) Get a good night's sleep. Sleeping disorders are commonly observed in people these days. If you are having trouble sleeping, you can always try peaceful techniques such as meditation and yoga. This will help you calm your nerve cells and will bring peace to a stressful mind. A reason why you might be going through a sleeping disorder can be food. If you relish a heavy and fatty meal at night just before sleeping, it will likely keep you up during the night and you will be making trips to the kitchen to drink water. The opposite is also true that if you did not have anything to eat before sleeping then a hungry stomach can also keep you awake at night. So, make sure to have a light and healthy snack before going to bed. Other helpful and researched techniques to get a better good night's sleep are to darken the room more and turn the face of the clock away from you. If you are worried about something, get the stress out of your mind and onto a piece of paper. It will not only provide your mind with a clearer perceptive but it will also help you feel peaceful because you can now quit worrying about it. If you have a habit of stressing too much about even little things, then meditation is necessary for you.

Exercise can also get the job done for you. Exercise tires out your body a little bit and when you lay down after it, you instantly feel peaceful and immediately go to sleep because of the tiredness factor.

So, here is one other benefit of daily exercise on top of a hundred others. Even after trying everything, you are unable to sleep soundly only then you should visit your doctor. Precaution is always better than medicine.

8) Avoid processed foods and sugars. Processed foods are unhealthy because they have already been deliberately changed before we consume them. Whenever the natural form of food is altered, it is categorized as 'processed'. You have always been hearing that eat fresh, eat healthily.

Minimally processed foods can retain their physical and nutritional properties. These include bagged salads, frozen vegetables, and meat. Then there comes some ready to eat foods.

You must know that they have been through ultra-processing, as they have been formulated from oils, fats, sugar, salt, added flavors, and preservatives. Always focus on eating fresh.

No matter what you eat, if it is fresh, it is much less likely to cause any harm to your stomach. Many beverages recently present in the market have a label of protein drinks, energy drinks, sports drinks, sugar-free drinks. All of these are a scam.

They have high amounts of added sugars and hundreds of different chemicals and substituents. Any drink that says 'sugar-free' means something else is added besides the sugar. Otherwise, the taste would be extremely bad and unbearable.

They can add artificial flavors or some other types of processed sugar and it can hurt your digestive system badly. Because instantly they will create a sugar high for you and when your sugar level drops back, you again crave it.

Continuous consumption of sugar can never do your body any good. Prefer fresh juices, fruit juices, and non-sugary beverages. Stay hydrated and let your body work at optimum levels.

9) Put away the salt shaker. A salt shaker at the dining table makes it too easy for you to consume excess salt. Excess salt can give you high blood pressure. So just pick the salt shaker up from the dining table and place it in a kitchen cupboard and only use it while preparing the meal. If you like spices or strong flavors in your food, you can add lime juice, garlic paste, or red pepper flakes.

Stock your fridge with fresh and dried herbs and use them instead of salt when needed. Blood pressure is the root cause of many different diseases and illnesses. It is also incurable.

People that have the problem of blood pressure have reported that it stays with you throughout your life. You have to daily eat a pill to keep your blood pressure at a normal level.

So, isn't it better that you avoid this problem altogether? Start eating meals with low amounts of salt and trust me, you will get used to the new taste in no time. It is not only healthy but also prevents you from spreading terminal and fatal diseases. Just satiate on the existing level of salt present in the dish or meal you are going to eat.

10) Give yourself a break. Believe it or not, overtraining can turn out to be a problem. If your body is not given enough time to restore, it won't restore its health and ultimately your performance will decline day by day instead of getting better.

Some symptoms help you know that you are overdoing it and those symptoms are; moodiness, constant fatigue, lack of energy, depression, and increased mental stress.

A common complaint heard from people is that "no matter how much I do cardio exercises; I cannot seem to lose more than I have lost already". It is because you are working out too much. Just take a short step back, give your body time to relax, and shorten your workout.

Another way to go around the problem is to divide and rule. If you do one hour of exercise, then divide it into two 30 minutes workout sessions; one in the morning and one in the evening.

This will prevent overtraining and will give your body time to rest in between. You can also start to work out on alternate days.

For example, if you had a work out on Monday, then skip the work out on Tuesday and have your next work out on Sunday. This will give time to your body that is enough for it to relax and restore its energy.

Always listen to what your body is telling you. Our bodies are well able to communicate with us, the problem do we listen or not.

How does Intermittent Fasting prevent cancer?

Intermittent Fasting helps to prevent cancer as well as it helps during its treatment. With each passing day, researches are being conducted on this matter and every day it proves further the fact that it does help in fighting cancer.

Prevention of cancer – Some research has shown that Intermittent Fasting fights cancer by lowering insulin resistance and levels of inflammation. Under the 'fasted state' of Intermittent Fasting, your body experiences lower insulin levels and tries to regain its energy by burning fats and excess calories.

As a result of this process, toxins and damaged cells present inside the body also get automatically burned. Naturally, we would never know that there any damaged cells present inside our body that can induce our bodies to cancer.

But Intermittent Fasting takes care of this problem on its own. It clears out all damaged and dysfunctional cells from our body which can later take shape of a tumor or cancer.

This provides prevention from cancer.

How does Intermittent Fasting help to treat cancer? Intermittent Fasting helps to boost the immune system which in return helps to fight cancer that is already present. Treatment of cancer needs the inner strength of the body so that it can fight it off. Intermittent Fasting provides the body with enough power and a stronger immune system and eventually, it overcomes the cancer cells.

Another way cancer can help treating Intermittent Fasting is during chemotherapy. Fasting makes cancer cells more responsive towards chemotherapy and this helps to protect the remaining cells of the body. During chemotherapy, Intermittent Fasting greatly helps in cellular regeneration. It also protects all cells and our blood from the side-effects of chemotherapy.

Chemotherapy has many other side-effects like fatigue, headaches, and nausea. Intermittent Fasting helps the body to deal with all these side-effects and helps to prevent them from happening.

So, for existing cancer patients, Intermittent Fasting can help them to tolerate the pain and ailment during fighting cancer. It helps them in overcoming side-effects and also gives the rest of their body protection from cancer. And those who have a family history of cancer and are susceptible to have cancer in the future are strongly recommended to intermittently fast.

This will help them with prevention from cancer. They will continuously keep getting rid of dangerous and dysfunctional cells and this greatly improves the chances of preventing those cells to take on a form of cancer.

IF makes healthy eating simpler and easier

The best diet is the one which you can stick to in the long-run. If Intermittent Fasting makes it easier and simpler for you to stick with a healthy diet plan then obviously you need to keep it as long as possible.

It will help you with maintaining a healthy weight and also helps you to remain in a healthy condition.

One of the main advantages of Intermittent Fasting is that it makes healthy eating simpler, easier, and less time-consuming.

Other diet plans may require you to tediously work out your carb intake and limit the calorie intake for the day. This is not practical. You cannot assess your meal every time before you eat it. That's how Intermittent Fasting takes the edge over dieting plans. It does not require you to limit your food choices and calorie intake.

It only helps you to maintain a healthy schedule of eating. Women who practice Intermittent Fasting, report that Intermittent Fasting helped them to move from 3 meals to 2 meals a day.

This made it easier for them to shift to a healthier lifestyle without drastically changing it. Intermittent Fasting limits the "feeding window" of the day to a few hours and this helps to move towards 2 meals a day plan. A gradual and steady shift in meals is important so that your body doesn't go into shock because of the new changes presented to it.

Start from 3 meals and then gradually progress towards two meals.

A diet is successful if it allows you to remain consistent and doesn't demand sudden lifestyle changes. So, in short, Intermittent Fasting is the best way to move to a healthier and easier lifestyle.

Chapter 6

Tips to ease through intermittent fast

Initially, you might find it hard to make it through the fast. It can be because you are not used to staying hungry. Researchers have put together a list of tips and strategies that will ease through the fasting cycle.

Suppress your hunger with the help of green tea, black coffee, and water. This is not a necessary step to implement during a fast; it's just for when you are experiencing an extreme hunger wave.

To satiate and suppress the hunger levels a little bit and ease through the fast; you can enjoy these drinks every once in a while.

Do not overdose on the amounts of these drinks and also don't drink them more than once or twice a day. Everything is bad when used in excess.

Try to listen and understand body cues. If you are feeling stress or anxiety without any significant reason, then it might be a cue from your body to relax. Feeling stressed in a fast is commonly observed especially during the initial days of fasting. This can often happen in certain periods of our lives.

This is not something to worry about but if it does not go away even after some time then it might be a signal from your body that it is getting exhausted.

Ease up on the hours of fasting and eat more nutrient-dense foods.

Have healthy food available in the house. Foods with protein and veggies should be available in your home all the time. In this way, when you break your fast on a Sunday evening, you should be able to have a small healthy meal at home.

Eating out is not prohibited in Intermittent Fasting. But every once in a while, have a home-prepared healthy and fresh diet. When you have available options at home, you will automatically be tempted to cook something delicious and healthy. Also, when you have healthy foods available at home, you will be much less tempted to go out and eat unhealthily.

Clean out your fridge to avoid temptation. It might be already hard for you to make it through the fast and if you know that chocolates and pizza are present inside your fridge, then the temptation can cross the limits. So before starting a fast, clean out temptations from your fridge so that your focus is diverted from what to eat now.

Eat meals after a fast relatively slower. You might be tempted to go out and eat a heavy and big meal after your first fast to celebrate. But this will make you feel so exhausted and lazy for the rest of the day that you won't be able to get out of bed.

So, a useful tip is to go slow while eating meals after a fast because it will help you to eat just enough and you will feel energized for the rest of your day.

Meditate and indulge in light exercise. Initially, your focus during a fast will just be food. You will keep counting how many hours you have to go more without food and this can induce stress in your brain. So, to take your attention off from thinking about food, start meditation. It will divert your attention as well as bring peace to your body and the rest of your day.

Light exercise helps to burn fat faster than anything. If your body allows you, then do indulge in light exercising. It will increase your physical fitness and will also increase the rate of weight-loss.

Eat plenty of whole foods on non-fasting days. Not everyone is looking to reduce weight through Intermittent Fasting.

Some people have a goal to get their body in a healthier condition than before. Even though fasting does involve staying away from foods for a certain portion of the day, it is still important to maintain a healthy eating style on the days when you are not fasting.

Eating healthy and whole foods will help you to stay away from all sorts of chronic illnesses as well as cancer. Whole foods include meat, eggs, fish, fruits, and vegetables.

Stop, if you are feeling unwell. Having a sick feeling or generally feeling unwell is a sign that fasting is not your thing. It can also mean that your body is not ready for fasting right now.

If you feel unwell or sick, then stop, focus on healthy eating, increase nutrition, and relax. Walk daily and slowly increase the time of walk so that your body can build higher stamina. Sometimes, you might have to help your body and this is one of those times.

Help your body to gain stamina and then when you feel healthy and energetic, you can try fasting again.

Re-evaluate your results. Try fasting for 7 days or 10 days before making a strong judgment call. You can try our 7-day guide that will help you make it through the initial 7 days of fasting.

After the specified time passes, if you still feel low on energy and a little light-headed then you need to ease up on fasting and choose another technique or formula of Intermittent Fasting. But if you feel great and active, then continue on your journey.

Research-proven advantages of IF for women

1) **Helps to regain hormonal balance.** Eating without any order and eating unhealthy can induce an imbalance of hormones inside your body. If because of any reason, you are having a hormonal imbalance and are looking for easy ways to restore the balance, then Intermittent Fasting is the way to go. Research has proven that Intermittent Fasting helps restore the eating order. It specifies the times of when to eat and when to stay hungry and it helps to maintain a healthy eating schedule. You may not realize the

importance of eating at regular times but the women who are having the problem of hormonal imbalance; should be asked about its importance. Just follow Intermittent Fasting and it will restore the balance of your hormones and will also take you to healthy eating schedules.

2) **Improves metabolism and insulin sensitivity.** Fasting induces low levels of insulin inside your body and when these levels are low; your body starts to gain energy from fats already present inside the body. So, higher insulin sensitivity means that your body easily goes to lower levels of insulin when fasting and thus starts to burn-off the fats. Another factor that contributes to the increase in insulin sensitivity in metabolic rate. If your metabolism is slow, you will be unable to digest the eaten meal quickly. It will take much longer for food to digest and thus won't give much time to your body to enter low insulin levels where it can burn-off fat. If you have a strong and fast metabolism, your body will process the food you ate much quicker, and your body will remain under low insulin levels for a higher time and thus burns a higher amount of fat. To increase your insulin sensitivity, research has proven that it is beneficial to indulge in Intermittent Fasting because it not only enhances your metabolism rate but also increases your body's sensitivity towards insulin levels.
3) **Improves eating patterns and hunger levels.** The research-proven best advantage of Intermittent Fasting is its power to improve eating patterns. Intermittent Fasting defines specific "eating periods" and "fasting periods". This helps to follow a timetable in eating. Eating at regular patterns has hundreds of proven benefits for the overall health of the body. It also helps with hunger levels. If you feel that you never really feel hungry, that means that you don't give time to your body to digest and have another meal before

the first one is digested. This causes adherence in entering fat-burning mode. You are eating regularly but you are not burning any fats. Fasting increases the hunger levels and helps your body to go into a fat-killing mode. Therefore, if you are experiencing problems related to eating patterns or hunger levels, indulge in moderate Intermittent Fasting.

4) **Effective for weight-loss.** Many kinds of research have been conducted on the important topic of "Does Intermittent Fasting help to lose weight or not?" You will be pleased to know that Intermittent Fasting is worldwide recognized as a weight-loss method. It not only helps you lose weight but it also helps you to maintain your health while doing so. Diets mostly leave people with different kinds of nutritional and physical deficiencies but Intermittent Fasting has been proven to have no such side-effects. Intermittent Fasting helps to increase insulin sensitivity which in return helps to lose weight because the body starts to burn the fats inside the body. When the fats are burned, the next time you have a meal; it is used to fulfill the needs of the body and is not just stored as fat. Higher the fat-burn, lower the fat-storage after the next meal and hence higher weight-loss.
5) **Improves brain function and makes the immune system stronger.** Intermittent Fasting has been proven to improve cognitive functions of the brain and make brain activity fast. When you eat at regular patterns and healthy, it provides healing powers to your entire body. The nutrition supplied helps to make all organs of the body to function better. Eating healthy and nutrition-dense foods help you to build a stronger immune system. The immune system has to fight-off all bacteria and diseases. If it's not healthy then it cannot provide your body the protection needed. Thus, to improve your immune system, you can opt for Intermittent Fasting.

6) **Fights diabetes and prevents cancer.** We already know that Intermittent Fasting helps with insulin sensitivity and keeps insulin levels at a lower rate than normal. This proves that Intermittent Fasting can greatly help patients with diabetes. It keeps the sugar levels at moderate levels; not too high or too low. It also helps with the prevention of cancer. Cancer is caused due to the storage of dysfunctional and harmful cells. These cells need to be taken out of the body and Intermittent Fasting greatly helps with it. When you fast, your body is in a fat-burning and harmful cell removal process. That's how Intermittent Fasting helps to prevent cancer. Improves cellular regeneration and discards harmful cells.
7) **Intermittent Fasting induces autophagy in your body.** Autophagy is a state in which the body itself clears out junk from your body. Here junk is referred for harmful and useless cells inside your body that need to be taken out. It not only clears out such cells from your body but also helps in the regeneration of new cells. Autophagy is a result of Intermittent Fasting. Without fasting, autophagy cannot be induced into the body naturally. Then you are left with chemotherapy only. So, to stay healthy and avoid medical procedures done on you, fast intermittently now and then.
8) **Engages your mind and body.** Some people have complained about constant stress in their minds. And they claim that there are no obvious reasons for the stress. Mental stress can be caused by one of many reasons. It can be due to a workaholic nature, not resting enough, not eating enough, not eating healthy, and never preparing healthy foods at home. Research has shown that when you fast for a specific time and then enjoy a nutritious meal afterward, it helps the brain to feel a sense of accomplishment. You will feel like you achieved something

out of your day and this provides satisfaction to your mind. Meanwhile, the body is already engaged in taking care of excess fats, burning extra calories, and sustaining its health and structure. Bu the end of the day, you will feel happy, enthusiastic, and much more energetic. Engaging the mind and body is necessary for a balanced body. So, Intermittent Fasting helps in another great way.

Reviews from women who practiced Intermittent Fasting

Surveys have been conducted and research has been undertaken to know about the reviews of women who practiced Intermittent Fasting. Reading these reviews can help you gain a clearer vision of what you can achieve by Intermittent Fasting, how did women successfully fasted, and did they face any problems or not.

The overall reviews were positive and women were highly appreciated and thanked for such a natural and easy to adopt technique. The reviews are listed below in the form of general information so that it's easy for you to read it and judge for yourself if it's something you can achieve too or not.

Women who tried Intermittent Fasting for a week

After one week of practicing it, women reported that they felt lighter. This doesn't mean they had a significant weight loss in a week.

It was just a way of expressing that they felt better and healthier than before. Some women said that weight-loss was little but negligible and some said they didn't have any weight-loss.

Again, these results were after just one week and the body takes this much time just to adjust to fasting schedules. They also reported about their appearance. One woman said that there was a loss of only a quarter of an inch around her waist and there were no other significant changes seen.

They also reported that by mid-week that is after 3 or 4 days of fasting, the dizziness and fogginess in their heads vanished due to fasting. And they didn't experience it anymore after that.

These women said that the biggest advantage of Intermittent Fasting that we observed in a week was that it was an extremely easy and simple technique to follow. It adjusts well with anybody's lifestyle and doesn't require any drastic changes either.

It not only helped them regulate their eating patterns but it also made them eat healthily. They said that Intermittent Fasting schedules made them try and enjoy nutrient-dense foods and that's why within a week, they experienced feeling lighter and healthier than before.

This proves that Intermittent Fasting promotes and makes it easy to regulate eating patterns as well as puts you in a habit of eating healthy. This increases your health and fitness on a huge scale in a very short time.

The woman who tried Intermittent Fasting for 8 months

A woman who tried Intermittent Fasting was asked about her experience and her results and she openly communicated them so that all the women out there can know about the long-term effects of Intermittent Fasting. Her experience is described below.

She said that after college she injured and fractured her foot which caused her to stop exercising and even moving at all.

That's why she started with Intermittent Fasting because she wanted to maintain a healthy and fit body even though she could not exercise. After 7.5 to 8 months, she dropped almost 50 pounds, around 10% body fat, and almost 40 inches all around her body.

And these were the results merely from intermittently fasting as she could do no walking or exercise. She was thankful for Intermittent Fasting because it helped her to get her BMI under the "normal' category, She said everybody asked her how she lost so much even when she could not exercise or walk.

She told everyone about her success due to Intermittent Fasting and also tried to bring them on this healthy technique too. She further said that the key to her success is Consistency.

She adopted the 4 days eat and 3-day fast schedule of Intermittent Fasting and never went any week without following this schedule.

The 3 days of fasting were non-consecutive and she made it clear many times. Women should not fast more than 24 hours and she followed the advice and it gained her the best possible results.

She had a little bit of difficulty in the starting week but this is something everyone faces. She saw that fasting had become easy for her before the first week even ended. So, this gives many tips and tricks for all the women out there. If you want the best results in a shorter time frame then there are a few things you need to consider.

First, find an Intermittent Fasting schedule suitable for you and stick to it. Second, you will have problems the first week like light-headedness or dizziness but don't worry; they will go away before or after one week.

Third, be consistent. Don't fast for one week and then stop fasting for the next week and then suddenly start fasting the week after that. This will induce an imbalance in your health, might even disturb your hormones and you will not be intrigued and willing to fast because your body is not being able to come under a habit of it. Whatever schedule you pick, stick with it, and stay consistent until the day you reach your goal weight.

Conclusion

Final words on Intermittent Fasting for women

Fasting is natural – humans have been doing it since forever.

The benefits of Intermittent Fasting greatly outweigh potential risks to it. These potential risks and dangers can only occur if you adopt a fasting lifestyle without having ample knowledge about how fasting works and what are important considerations to keep in mind.

To be further safe, you can also ask your doctor if it is healthy for you to fast or not.

If you are not suffering from a chronic disease or specific medical conditions, then your doctor is most likely to give you the "go-ahead".

Intermittent Fasting is a technique with various formulas. And you can try and adapt any of these formulas according to your lifestyle and preferences.

You can take benefit from its many advantages like weight-loss, disease prevention, better mental and physical performance, and overall fitness and health. Intermittent Fasting allows you to choose your fasting and feeding windows so that your body can optimally work and also meet its calorie needs.

One picture of Intermittent Fasting that you don't want to be in is – you fast for 24 hours and then satisfy your hunger with binge-eating.

You also don't want to exceed the 24 hours specifies limit for women. Fasting is worth it because it will give you mental clarity in the morning before going to work. It does not affect your lifestyle.

You can exercise according to your own desired intensity. You will sleep better and faster. And most important above all; you will lose a healthy amount of weight without it paralyzing your health!

Before getting started, try different schedules of fasting. Eat normally and then fast 1 or 2 times a week. Or fast and feast regularly in a day. Or fast every other day occasionally.

Try out all these options before settling down with one formula of Intermittent Fasting.

Ease into Intermittent Fasting by starting from short fasting and eating windows. It will help you with initial hunger and discomfort. But if it becomes too uncomfortable, be honest with yourself and just take a step back!

At the end of the day, nothing can have a greater impact on your health than a lifestyle that prioritizes your mental, physical, and emotional well-being. And a nutrition style that comprises real whole foods, not just empty carbs.

No diet can offer you all of this in one package. But Intermittent Fasting is a gift for you with everything complimentary.

Intermittent Fasting for Women

Written by Jenna Dawson

First Edition

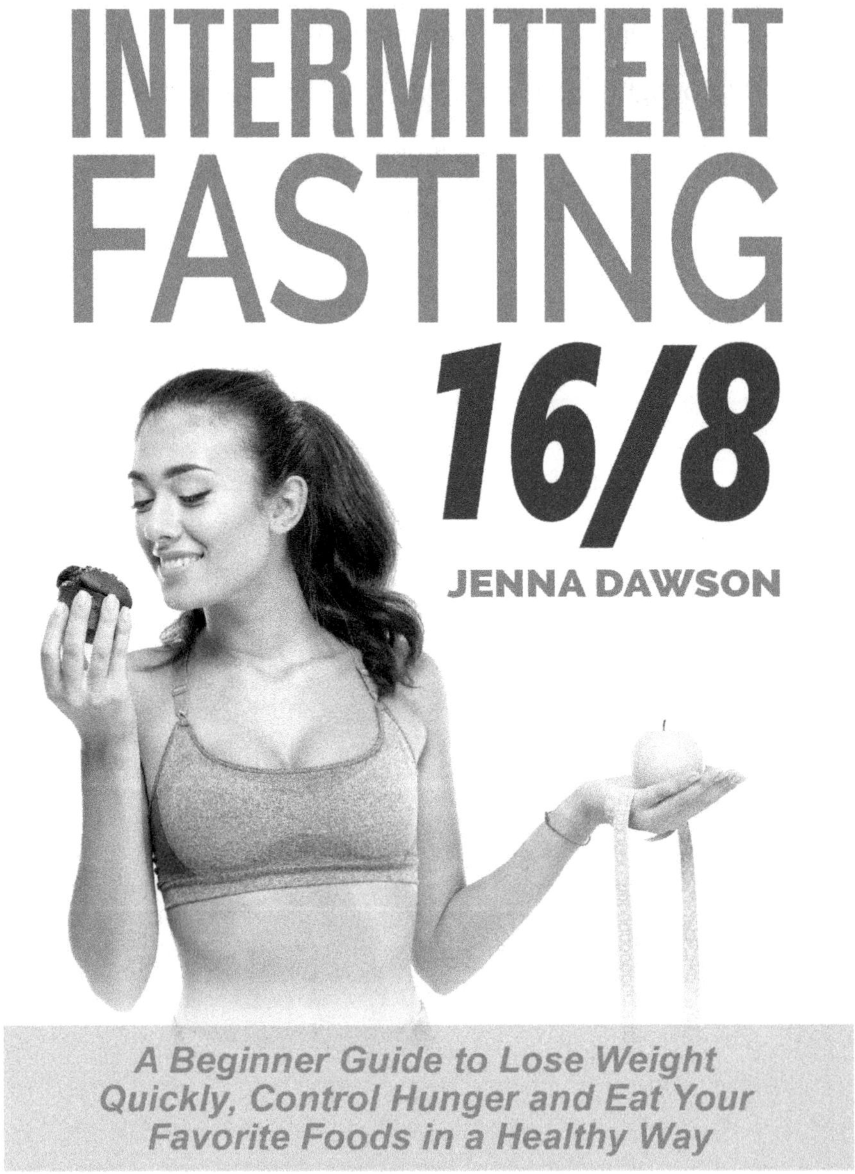
INTERMITTENT
FASTING
16/8
JENNA DAWSON
A Beginner Guide to Lose Weight
Quickly, Control Hunger and Eat Your
Favorite Foods in a Healthy Way

page intentionally left blank

Intermittent Fasting 16/8

A Beginner Guide to Lose Weight Quickly, Control Hunger and Eat Your Favorite Foods in a Healthy Way

Jenna Dawson

Intermittent Fasting 16/8

Written by Jenna Dawson

First Edition

Copyrights Notice

Limited Liability

Please note that the content of this book is based on personal experience and various information sources. Although the author has made every effort to present accurate, up-to-date, reliable, and complete information in this book, they make no representations or warranties concerning the accuracy or completeness of the content of this book and specifically disclaim any implied warranties of merchantability or fitness for a particular purpose.

Your particular circumstances may not be suited to the example illustrated in this book; in fact, they likely will not be. You should use the information in this book at your own risk.

All trademarks, service marks, product names, and the characteristics of any names mentioned in this book are considered the property of their respective owners and are used only for reference. No endorsement is implied when we use one of these terms.

This book is only for personal use. Please note the information contained within this document is for educational and entertainment purposes only and no warranties of any kind are declared or implied. Readers acknowledge that the author is not engaged in providing medical, dietary, nutritional, or professional advice, or physical training.

Please consult a doctor, nutritionist or dietician, before attempting any techniques outlined in this book. Nothing in this book is intended to replace common sense or medical consultation or professional advice and is meant only to inform. By reading this book, the reader agrees that under no circumstances is the author responsible for any losses, direct or indirect, which are incurred as a result of the use of the information contained within this document, including, but not limited to, errors, omissions, or inaccuracies.

Table of Contents

Introduction....144

Chapter 1....146

How Intermittent Fasting 16/8 Works....147

Chapter 2....152

Getting Started....153

Appropriate 16/8 Time Frame and Period....154

Best foods to eat during the Eating Window....159

Number of meals to be taken in a day....163

Chapter 3....166

What to eat and drink during your Eating Window....167

Managing the Macronutrients....170

Three-Stage Process for 16/8 Intermittent Fasting Protocol....172

You will need to manage....175

Chapter 4....178

Suitable people to go for Intermittent Fasting 16/8....179

Intermittent Fasting for Women....183

16/8 Intermittent Fasting for Men....187

Chapter 5....192

Intermittent Fasting and your metabolism....193

1 - Fasting and the brain....194

2 - Burns fat for fuel....195

3 - Boosts your energy....195

4 - Boosts HIGH Levels....195

Muscle mass and Intermittent Fasting 196
Chapter 6 198
Strategies for losing weight quickly 199
To maintain weight with Intermittent Fasting 16/8 .... **Error! Bookmark not defined.**
Benefits of exercise 208
The best exercise to enhance the advantages of Fasting....... 210
Chapter 7 212
Mistakes to avoid committing.. 213
Intermittent Fasting myths 220
Chapter 8 226
Side effects of Intermittent Fasting 227
Sample routine 230
30 Days Meal-Plan to help you while on IF 16/8 239
Hacks to help you succeed.. 247
Conclusion 256

Introduction

This is the easiest type of fasting if you have never tried intermittent fasting. This is the most popular time. The eating window is within eight hours and your fasting window is 16 hours in the day. This can be flexible, and you can attain similar benefits from either skipping breakfast or dinner.

If you are just beginning to embrace intermittent fasting in your life, begin slowly and try skipping a meal. See if you can plan towards a 16-hour fast and 8-hour eating window.

Fasting Within a Daily Window

There are various other eating windows you can implement like the 16:8 method. You already fast to some extent between your evening dinner and the next morning's breakfast.

This is what you can do to adjust the eating/fasting windows:

Eat your breakfast at 9 am with your last meal of the day at 6 pm.

You ate within a 9-hour window. Your fasting window will be 15 hours. The next step is to widen your intermittent fasting window and have a narrower eating window. Another 16:8 method could be when you eat your meals between 10 am to 6 pm.

Chapter 1

How Intermittent Fasting 16/8 Works

One thing that you should know about intermittent fasting is that you can't consider it as a diet plan. It is an eating pattern, which requires you to schedule your meals to maximize their positive effects on your fitness and health. The pattern involves a cycle composed of separate periods of eating and fasting.

So basically, this eating pattern does not require you to change the foods you eat. What you need to change is you're eating schedule.

Now, you may be asking yourself if it is worthwhile to make some changes to when you should eat. The answer is a resounding yes.

IF is an incredible solution if you want to be lean and stay that way without having to follow crazy and difficult diet plans or focus too much on counting calories. In most cases, this eating pattern even requires you to retain your calorie intake when you are still starting.

Besides, it is a great way of preserving your muscle mass while still keeping your body lean. It is also the simplest strategy if you want to take off unwanted weight and ensure that you stay within your target. You can do that without making excessive changes in your behavior. This makes intermittent fasting simple and doable in the sense that anyone can easily do it while remaining meaningful as it truly creates a positive difference in your weight and health.

All our lives we heard our parents say, "Breakfast is the most vital meal of the day!", but are they right?

It's an awful tip, suggest the Leangains, the popular 16/8 hour method. With the Leangains, Martin Berkhan introduced the skipping of breakfast, extending the fasting period, and taking advantage of the natural fast during sleeping hours.

The plan is to fast overnight and the first 6 hours of the day making a total of 16 hours, then eating all your calories in the remaining 8 hours. For example; suppose you woke up at 6 am, waited for the next 6 hours until midnight, and from 12 pm to 8 pm you get to eat all your carbohydrates and proteins as large, fulfilling meals. You make this way of eating pattern your lifestyle, and the results are obvious.

Why skip breakfast is what you are wondering, right? The idea of 'skipping a morning meal is bad for you' began with studies sponsored by cereal companies to increase sales.

This powerful message has been transferred on and has been engraved in the minds of people for so many years that it has become a proper belief. Now imagine... After taking your last meal, you fell asleep, and you woke up to a very low insulin level.

Trust me, the worst thing you can do to yourself right now would be having a high carbohydrate diet which will eventually increase your insulin level, depositing fat stores, and shutting the fat burning process for nothing less than 12 hours minimum. Also, this will soon bring the hunger growls in the stomach as the high insulin levels will result in low glucose levels.

Extension of fasting in the 16/8 process does wonders by triggering the metabolic phase, shifting the energy metabolism more on ketones than on glucose. This time-restricted feeding can also decrease the abnormalities linked to obesity.

During the 6 hours fast, you can have all the no-calorie liquids, the most important being mineral water. However, the water intake is advised best at certain times. Similarly, snacking is allowed during the fed state, but it's better to have three full meals than nibbling all the time.

Have healthy food with more veggies, fruits, fiber, and protein, but no sugars and no snacking. This will give your body a rest and time to digest the food by breaking it and using it as energy photons to keep you active during the day.

This brings in the significance of exercise or at least staying active in the IMF (Intermittent Fasting) 16/8. If you cannot go to the gym, do weight lifting exercises such as pushups or squats at home.

What matters is that you are not sitting idle. You can go swimming or to a park for cardio such as jogging or brisk walk. Fasting alone might burn your fat, but it will not help you achieve the desired goal. If we do not use the energy stored in our bodies, then our bodies end up storing this energy as fat, making us lazy.

Therefore, exercise is vital for your general well-being, health, mental, and physical strength and it will also lighten your mood.

No doubt it worked for the bodybuilders, since the IMF 16/8 slows down the muscle tearing process, unlike in other diet programs, thus this is where its fame began. The weight loss encountered by the bodybuilders was tremendous, and the muscle growth was the best part. Many people have the wrong perception that fasting leads to burning muscle instead of burning fat.

However, this is not true. Instead, it activates the growth hormone. The hormone in combination with testosterone burns fat and consequently builds as much muscle as it can. It also keeps us focused and increases our level of alertness.

Researches have shown that the 16 hours fast does nothing unhealthy, but improves the body in every way possible. In fact, in 2014, research Mattson wrote that, fasting for 16 hours a day sets in motion the stress adjustment medium, which offers immunity against disorders and diseases.

Varady, the associate professor, talks about the latest study at the University of Illinois, in which the researchers worked with 23 obese volunteers with the IMF 16/8 method. The average age of the volunteers was about 45. It took them about 12 weeks after which the results were chosen for comparison with other fasting methods. Although the results were highly similar to previous reports from other fasting methods with insulin sensitivity and weight loss, the volunteers for them consumed fewer calories.

However, he was surprised to see the weight maintenance the 16/8 program had shown. It was also less tough than the other methods, which followed the low number of dropouts from the experiment. People themselves have to figure out what works best for them, and therefore the famous quote goes, "Work hard in silence, and let the success do its talking".

We have been talking about low insulin levels and better insulin sensitivity, but how is it good? Why should people aim for it, after all? The Journal of Physiology presented a study related to better insulin sensitivity and low insulin levels after weight loss and workouts. The role of the study was to determine the effects of weight loss and training on the body.

There were two kinds of research conducted, one with the exercise and the other without exercise. Both resulted in a weight loss of about 12% and improved insulin sensitivity by approximately 60%.

However, the oxidative capacity increased by 25% with the exercise. This indicated that increasing the oxidative capacity through exercise does not affect insulin sensitivity as the main indicator is weight loss.

If you can lose weight, your insulin sensitivities will stay in control, especially in obese men and women, but again why do we need to increase our insulin sensitivity?

Insulin resistance is an omnipresent metabolic problem linked to obesity. Insulin is a peptide hormone secreted by the pancreatic Islets of Langerhans which maintains blood glucose levels. The adipose tissues and muscle insulin plays an important role in weight loss.

In the muscles, during the fed state, insulin encourages glycogen synthesis through the stimulation of glycogen synthase. To enable energy to be anaerobically released through glycolysis, this activation is necessary, for example, during an intense muscular workout. Muscle cells are not dependent on glucose or glycogen for energy release during the basal state when insulin levels are low. Therefore, low insulin levels divert the attention from burning glucose to finding other sources of energy, and this helps in building muscles as well as weight loss. Low insulin levels also promote the catabolism of protein which is not healthy.

Starvation motivates this breakdown of protein molecules, while a diet routine with intermittent fasting done in the right terms and conditions, does not let the body reach this state.

Chapter 2

Getting Started

You should always remember that! Intermittent fasting is not a diet. It is more of a routine than a diet plan, thus once you decide to go for IMF the next step to make is what your fasting and eating time frames will be. Does this mean that you are restricted to a time window? Well, that's where this becomes interesting.

The ideal part is that not only do you get to choose the time window yourself, but you can also adjust it according to your comfort zone.

The only thing to be taken care of is that you need to complete your fasting hours. You need to see which meals you are comfortable skipping and how well you'll be able to adjust to skipping them. You can consider your routine with work timings, school timings, etc. This point is like a bonus to the routine.

Let's check your daily activities to fit in the 16/8 hours. Most people prefer starting their fast around bedtime so that half of their fast passes while they are sleeping. They can skip breakfast as part of the fast and have lunch and dinner during their eating window.

You follow your time frame according to the routine every day, but what if you are employed and have to work all day, or maybe you are a late-night freak that wakes up late, or you have weekend plans to catch up with your squad?

It's pretty simple! If skipping breakfast isn't an option for you, you can adjust your eating window earlier in the day around 8 a.m. to 4 p.m. If you wake up late, you automatically skip breakfast and keep a night fast. If you have weekend plans such as late-night dinners with friends and family, you straight away shift your fasting window earlier or during the time you are free.

These are just examples of how you can adjust your eating window to suit your own eating needs and habits. During your eating window, you must fill yourself up strategically so that you do not get hungry during your fast, and you can even change your eating window every day according to your workload. However, it's best to keep a fixed window and only change it in cases of emergencies, because as human being our urge for food comes with the daily pattern we set for ourselves, and breaking the pattern every day will not only be confusing but will also be inconvenient. Anyways, ensure having a healthy diet.

Appropriate 16/8 Time Frame and Period

The fasting window can be adjusted according to the meal skipping schedule:

- skip breakfast: eat lunch and dinner;
- skip lunch: eat breakfast in the morning, start your fast, and enjoy dinner;
- skip dinner: eat breakfast and lunch and go for an overnight fast

A similar study was conducted at the University of Alabama on a group of men with prediabetes. They also practiced the time-restricted feeding, but at an earlier time frame.

The 8-hour period started at 7 am and ended at 3 pm, with all the meals fitting in the time duration. Although there were no signs of weight loss, after 5 weeks both the groups had eye-catching low insulin levels and their insulin sensitivity had also improved amazingly. According to the volunteers, they did not starve although it was tough at the beginning. Later, they noticed a remarkable and controlled decrease in their appetite.

While making sure that your decision of choosing IMF is right, you need to do things accurately. As a beginner, start with baby steps and do not rush yourself. Although the breathtaking results of others might have excited you and you want similar results as soon as possible, just think how they all started. The start must build your stamina rather than breaking it. Learn from the mistakes and experiences of others, even those who dropped out.

"Rome wasn't built in one day, but they worked on it every single day!", and this is how the fasting process operates entirely. A 16-24 hour fast is not a norm for a human being who has to go to work every day, do the chores at their homes, take care of their children, and stay active. We do not advise you to underestimate yourself but give time to your body to adapt to the changes in such a way that it causes no harm physically and mentally.

A median American is accustomed to feed themselves self in a 12-hour cycle, with a 12 hour fast which includes sleeping. This makes them pretty much adapted to the minimum fasting requirement of IMF. Similarly, fasting in many religions has a religious value to people, and therefore they are used to fasting for a month annually.

Considering a person who has never fasted before, it can be tough for them especially looking at other factors such as their age, height, mass, and food preferences.

They need to set up a period to start with. This will eventually lend the body and cells time to conquer the hunger pangs. The insulin and energy sensitivities will start to store energy for longer periods and to lower insulin to switch from glucose to fat burning.

IMF is simple once you get the hang of it, but before you get the hang of it you must go through the tough times.

Make intermittent fasting 16/8 your lifestyle. Once in the zone, and when your body is comfortable with the procedure, "fast more, feed less," and let the words repeat in your mind like a drill to keep the pattern.

There is no uncertainty on the fact that the longer the fast, the more effectively it functions and the sooner is the fruit visible, but as we mentioned before, don't be restless.

Between trying and triumph, be the "umph" in the triumph! The extended restraining periods would not harm you, until and unless you are providing your body with what it wants during the eating window. Consistency is going to be of more value than the time frame of your feeding window.

Moving on to how long the drill is preferred to be continued. If you are a beginner, you need to know whether the process goes well with your body, so it is recommended to try the fast weekly or every three weeks, and if you do not face issues of any sort then continue.

Later on, as your two initial weeks are over and you approach the third and fourth week, you start monitoring everything. Adjust your sleep in such a way that you are done eating at least three hours before bedtime. This is because our brain has a nucleus that syncs in our sleeping patterns, dreams, and metabolism through the light that enters our retina.

Now we can imagine how late-night browsing on our laptops, iPads, and mobiles, snacking and heavy meals can stray our internal clocks. It also creates confusion between our brain and body since the brain wants to rest and the body full of energy is ready to burn. The best way to stop the functioning of your peripheral clocks is to stop eating at 7 pm.

It is time to tighten up as we enter the fifth and sixth weeks of time-restricted feeding. You shift the eating window to exactly 8 to 9 hours. By this time, you must have learned to make good food choices. You can continue eating the food that you have been eating, just cut down on the sugar.

You could try to incorporate coconut oil in your cooking and add more fish, or fish oil, into your diet. Now is the time where you start shredding your excess fat. The adipose fatty tissue burns, reducing the symptoms of obesity, and improving the quality of life.

The eating window describes your lifestyle. Fasting improves your lifestyle to the extent that it reduces the risk of breast cancer in women by 40%. Also, this is irrespective of the food eaten. Isn't it incredible? Further weeks lead to longer fasting and their effects.

Before giving up, glue yourself to it for at least a month, unless you face a medical condition.

Do not think of the outcome only in terms of the needle going down the scale. If the results are positive, the needle on the scale will go up due to muscle build-up, the digestion will get better, and so will you sleep, making you feel good.

By the end of the acclimation period, you'll know whether intermittent fasting is a good fit for you or not and whether you can handle it. There's no better teacher than experience.

Good health is an endless journey. As long as we are alive, good health should always remain our goal. However, when we start our journey towards good health, it is always important to set milestones to gauge our progress. Milestones help in judging the progress, and also give us an insight for course correction.

Unlike other weight loss measures, intermittent fasting is not linear. It has a wide scope. People practice intermittent fasting for various objectives.

People follow intermittent fasting for 3 main purposes:

1) Losing Weight and Burning Fat
2) Maintaining the Current Weight
3) Holistic Health

You can be practicing intermittent fasting for any of these goals, but you can't judge the progress with the same scale.

It's very important to set benchmarks for progress to ensure that the methods are working for you. Your goals must also be in line with the kind of effort you are putting in. If you are putting in a lot of effort, and yet you are not getting the results, then you would need to do course correction. Intermittent Fasting for Burning Fat and Losing Weight. This is one of the most popular goals, as people these days are struggling with weight issues.

There are two ways to judge progress in this area.

1) You should measure the target areas like the waistline, hips, and thighs with a measuring tape to see if the fat-burning is taking place.
2) You should weigh yourself on the scale to see if the weight is going down.

There can be any one of the following scenarios:

1) Your weight is going down, but your waistline remains the same. This happens in the first few weeks of beginning intermittent fasting. Your weight may drop drastically as the body starts dumping a lot of water. You must have patience as the body would start burning fat very soon.
2) You are losing weight as well as your waistline is also going down. This usually happens in the beginning phases, and your body loses weight as well as burns fat too.
3) Your waistline is going down, but your weight is not going down. This can happen when your body burns fat, but also starts building muscles. The muscles are compact and have more weight. Therefore, you may not see any significant change in your weight on the scale. However, this is a positive thing.

If your observation is something different, then you would need to revisit the whole process and determine the point where you are making a deviation of mistake.

Intermittent Fasting for Weight Maintenance. Maintenance of the existing weight is also a goal people have these days, and it is a very important thing. If the weight starts growing uncontrollably, the day is not far when you will be surrounded by several diseases. Therefore, you must get a weight bracket for yourself. You can make changes in your diet and workout routines whenever you notice any significant change in your weight bracket or the waistline.

Intermittent Fasting for Improving Overall Health. Improvement of overall health is a goal everyone must-have. If you are healthy, the accumulation of fat is the last thing to happen. Your body is always capable of fighting all the excesses. To judge health improvement, you will need to take some tests before beginning intermittent fasting, and then keep repeating them at regular intervals.

Best foods to eat during the Eating Window

Intermittent fasting is one of the key solutions for your body to clean out and repair any cellular junk that you have accumulated for several years. This results in the improved function of your body organs and systems.

However, you can't expect this eating pattern to perform such an important role successfully if you do not support it with adequate amounts of nutritious foods. The right foods are essential in the process of replenishing and rebuilding your body.

You have to pick whole and good foods with high nutrient density. Eventually, your body will master the art of signaling when it already had enough food. In return, you will also master the art of listening to your body cues. This will allow you to eat less than what you normally consume before without being too restrictive.

Another thing that you have to remember about intermittent fasting is that it will not work if you follow an extremely restrictive diet. It is because this might cause you to be extremely starved physically and emotionally. This might result in you overeating due to deprivation, so avoid making yourself feel too hungry unnecessarily for a long period.

Just make sure to avoid sticking to processed and unhealthy foods. You still need a well-balanced diet rich in whole and nutritious foods for intermittent fasting to help you in reaching your weight loss and health goals.

So, what are the best foods to eat during your eating window? Here are some of the most nutritious ones:

Whole Grains – Carbs are vital for your health. You can't consider them as your mortal enemy when trying to lose weight. Note that since you are practicing intermittent fasting, a huge chunk of your daily routine will be spent on the fasted state.

With that in mind, you need to look for a strategic solution to obtain enough calories without overeating. Yes, you will need to minimize processed foods but you can also include some from time to time, like whole-grain bread, crackers, and bagels.

It is because your body can quickly digest these foods, giving you a good supply of fuel in an instant. They also serve as excellent sources of energy if you are training or exercising regularly while doing the fast. What is good about whole grains is that they also have high amounts of protein and fiber. This means that you do not have to eat too much of it to keep yourself full.

It is also advisable to eat whole grains instead of refined ones as the former can improve your metabolism. Among the healthiest whole grains that you can include in your diet to further improve the results of IF are amaranth, sorghum, millet, spelled, and bulgur.

- Lentil – This is a highly nutritious food, which is rich in fiber. One-half cup of it can already provide up to 32% of the total amount of fiber you need every day. Aside from fiber, lentil is also rich in iron, which is good if you are an active female who is also trying to stick to intermittent fasting.
- Potatoes – Just like bread, potatoes can also be digested by your body with the least amount of effort. Pairing it with a

good source of protein can turn it into a great post-workout snack designed to refuel your hungry and tired muscles. Another advantage of including potatoes in your regular diet if you are following the intermittent fasting approach is that they are effective in forming a resistant starch, which can fuel the good bacteria present in your gut.

- Nuts – While the calorie content of nuts is higher compared to other snacks, they are still good for your body because they have an important component not present in the majority of junk foods – that is good fat. You can take advantage of the polyunsaturated fat present in walnut to change the physiological markers linked to both satiety and hunger, making this snack beneficial for intermittent fasters.
- Eggs – Even one piece of large egg already contains up to 6 grams of protein, which helps make yourself feel full as well as in the muscle-building process. Another advantage of eggs is that they are easy and quick to prepare. They are ready within just a few minutes. Hard-boiled eggs are also both filling and nutritious, making them perfect additions to your eating window.
- Berries – Different kinds of berries can also help fill you up while providing your body with essential nutrients. Strawberries, for instance, are excellent sources of Vitamin C, which can boost your immunity. You can also eat blueberries that have high flavonoid content. There are also fiber-rich raspberries that are great additions to your diet. Note that each cup of raspberries already contains 8 grams of fiber, keeping you full and regular even during your shortened eating window.
- Fish – Intermittent fasting can produce even better results for you if you include fish in your eating schedule. Aside from having high protein and healthy fat content, different

kinds of fish are also rich in Vitamin D. It provides a sufficient amount of nutrients, which is great if your food intake will be limited only to your eating window. What's good about fish is that it is also considered as brain food, which is great during the times when you are restricting your calorie intake that might affect your cognition.

- Cruciferous Vegetables – These include cauliflower, Brussels sprouts, and broccoli – all of which have high fiber content. Note that erratic eating caused by adapting the intermittent fasting approach to weight loss requires you to consume more fiber-rich foods to avoid constipation and keep you regular. What is great about fiber is that it also leads to fullness, which is beneficial especially if you are planning to go through the day with most hours spent on fasting.
- Legumes and beans – Adapting to the IF lifestyle might prompt you to fall in love with legumes and beans that are rich in low-calorie carbs that can supply you with enough energy for your daily activities. This makes them vital additions to your eating plan. Also, foods that belong to the legume and bean family including black beans, lentils, peas, and chickpeas can significantly reduce your body weight even if you do not restrict your calorie intake.

Following the intermittent fasting lifestyle can indeed give you desirable results but you have to make sure that you are also helping yourself by eating the right foods. Make sure that when you break the fast, your focus is on foods rich in essential vitamins and protein.

These nutrients are necessary for boosting your immunity. It also helps to add fiber-rich foods into your eating plan to ensure that your digestive system continues to work properly. Go for olive oil, tomatoes, oily fish, and nuts.

You should also know what foods to stay away from. Avoid refined carbs, including chips, cakes, biscuits, and sugar as your body might convert these foods to fat quickly. If you wish to eat foods with a lower calorie content than usual then ensure that the calories are as nutritious and as good for your body as possible.

Note that just because you need to eat calories does not mean that you should get these calories from low-quality and unhealthy sources.

Number of meals to be taken in a day

There is a common myth about how eating small frequent meals is good for health. We are going to bust this myth right here, right now! Throughout times, information can get distorted for many reasons, and this is one of those cases.

We have listened to value less advice in abundance all our lives, and this has been one of them. The myth says to run your body's metabolism by continuously feeding yourself, having 6 to 8 small meals instead of 3 full meals. This will keep you active, energetic, prevent your sugar level from falling, and will keep you away from the starvation mode. How do you tend to believe this without any evidence? The truth is the other way round.

In a 2005 study, Mattson wrote about the results of meal frequency on human well-being. 2 years later in 2007, Stote had the results of other scientific studies published regarding how the calorie intake in humans differed and affected the anatomy in one versus three meal intakes. The calories in one meal per day were equal to the calories of the three meals.

The results were significantly the same in terms of blood pressure, heart rate, and even the optimal body temperature; however, there was a slight increase in blood pressure with the one-day meal. This was explained by the doctors themselves as they had taken the results for both experiments at different time durations.

The fact supporting the argument was that the same experiment done on mice had a decrease in blood pressure and a normal heart rate.

The author's explanation for this contradiction of results was that the circadian rhythms influence on human and animal blood pressure had differences. The final verdict of the study was that even in the absence of calorie restriction, the consumption of only one meal leads to not only more weight loss, but also a tremendous decrease in the mass of adipose tissue.

The effects on mice also lead to the conclusion that the application of intermittent fasting 16/8 in the absence of calorie restriction proved to be effective for decreasing abnormalities related to obesity.

Reviewing the studies, an article supported with little evidence suggested that gastro patients follow the 6 meals pattern to which the responses of other authors were not at all encouraging. The side effects of this included weight gain issues, sleep deprivation, and eating disorders.

Clearing out the mixed perceptions on the number of meals per day, brings us back to the point of how skipping breakfast will contribute to a lesser number of meals and what effects it will have?

Chowdhary and his colleagues carried a 6 week trial in obese individuals. The effects of the no breakfast group were compared with the control group. The one day trial showed symptoms of hunger in the individuals with a prolonged day fast with high plasma levels, high glucose, and insulin levels post-lunch.

Contrarily, individuals on their breakfast day had low leptin, acetylated ghrelin levels, but on both days, there was no effect on the calorie intake. Interestingly, there was no change in any results after the 6 weeks controlled trial in both the breakfast and non-breakfast meal days.

Looking at IMF 16/8, meal frequency is a matter of one's liking, and if we are taking the right food at the right time or not? In the end, it all comes to what makes you comfortable and responds best to your body. After reading the T-Nation article by Brad Schoenfeld, the meal frequency issue gets all sorted in your mind.

Although talking about our energy level in practical life, the 6 meals in a day may sound logical, but the total calories burned remain constant as there is no difference in thermogenesis.

The study by the American Journal was designed over two 8-weeks periods. Individuals were supposed to consume all the calories in either 3 meals or 1 meal. If they maintained their body weight within 2 kilograms, they enjoyed the benefits of body composition including body mass reductions.

The individuals who were able to adjust to one meal had to face increased hunger and were also supposed to take appropriate calories or else they had to face adverse effects.

The three meals can be adjusted in your daily life pretty easily, according to Justin's article. The hunger sensation can ultimately lead you to over-eat later, so you need to take care of that.

Do not pick and choose from the routine when going for intermittent fasting, because it does not work that way.

Chapter 3

What to eat and drink during your Eating Window

The eating window has to be everyone's favorite segment of the day. This is because it is restriction-free! Yes, you are allowed to eat absolutely anything during this 8-hour duration. You do not have to stare at the tempting and mouthwatering cupcakes from behind the refrigerator glass and control yourself.

Since you are building up your resistance level, and saving calories during day fasts, you have nothing to worry about. Do not be guilty of having that cheesy thin-crust pizza or a juicy beef burger or a delicious dessert, because you deserve it. However, if you want that Rihanna figure and want the results to show sooner, you will have to give up on some calories. What's best is to shift to a healthy diet providing you all the nutrients that will keep the energy alive during the fasting state.

Start your feast state with plenty of water around half an hour before having your meal, as it helps during digestion. In your meals include high protein content. By a high protein meal, we mean that having it once a day is enough. The protein will shrink your appetite and increase the number of calories you burn with a high metabolic rate. These burned calories can make up to 80 to 100 calories a day. It can also help you to maintain your weight in the long run with minimal effort.

Avoid any sugary items, including fruit juices and sodas. This modern way of added sugar in liquids is the most fattening of all as our brain does not recognize the liquid fat in the same way as the solid form. Prefer eating fiber-rich carbohydrates to refined ones. Note that carbohydrates instantly convert to glucose and that your body prefers glucose breakdown for energy before any other source.

Keep yourself hydrated all the time, and drink plenty of water. Yes, you can have tea and coffee even after the eating window, but without sugar. If you are skipping breakfast, tea or black coffee is just it. How easy is that? No rushing to grab breakfast on your way or any hassle of cooking early in the morning. An early morning black coffee will make you alert with the extra caffeine it has, but do not use cream or milk, or sugar. We know getting used to black coffee can be hard, but you have no alternative. Although if you think you might die without that splash of cream, then use it, but try and keep usage minimal. You can also consider having detox drinks such as warm water with one whole squeezed lemon and honey. This is a famous detox drink that individuals have on an empty stomach in, early morning. Similarly, green tea after meals can highly contribute to the success rate of weight loss. All of this depends on your preferences and diet chart, which may also have yogurt, protein shakes, and smoothies.

You can minimize the number of calories naturally too by eating food with maximum nutrient density at minimal quantities during the eating window. These include meat, fish, dairy items, fruits, and nuts. Adding avocados to your diet can be wonderful. We know that you must be thinking that despite it being the highest calorie food, why are we recommending it. Well, a study in a Nutrition Journal proves that adding even half an avocado to your meal can keep you full for hours, longer than you can imagine. Along with potatoes, it is one of the most satiating foods ever. Foods like black beans and chickpeas can result in weight loss even without calorie restriction. Also, consider adding pro-biotic items to your meals to avoid any kind of unpleasantness or discomfort like constipation.

Did you know that a recent study in correspondence with Harvard had found out that people who had berries such as raspberries, blueberries, and strawberries along with their meals, had a low body mass index increase when compared to individuals who ate no berries at all? Finally, eggs are rich in protein and reduce your hunger pangs. A study suggests that people who prefer eggs over bagels stay less hungry over their daily schedule.

What about chewing gums? You can have them during your eating window, but not during the fast, especially if they are not sugar-free. In the case of sugar-free gums, they have 2 to 3 calories only, but it's better to avoid them as they are unhealthy.

Do not forget that you are exercising along with a 16/8 hour routine, and you need to be full of energy. When you have your high resistance training days, make sure to add carbohydrates to your basic diet plan. Even with normal training, keep your meals healthy and add high-density nutrient foods to keep your energy level up and to avoid fatigue. After training, keep your water drinking cycle on point, and have your biggest meal then. Having your biggest meal right after exercise will boost up your metabolism, and keep you mobile. Remember that intermittent fasting alone, without any physical fatigue is not as effective as it can be.

The more you stress out on the routine, the more you mess up, so relax. IMF is just as simple as it sounds. Decide for yourself a time frame and period that suits you, and then just go with the flow.

Wake up, fast, eat, and sleep, or do it the other way round. It does not matter! What you do during IMF 16/8, is all in front of you, clear as crystal. How do you prefer doing it is your own choice. You are not moving away from your daily routine, just improving it for your health.

The reason behind the success of this intermittent fasting protocol is its long-term sustainability. It is so easy to follow that you can continue with this routine effortlessly without having to think about it. This means that you can follow it for years without having to take a break. This intermittent fasting protocol not only helps you in losing weight and burning fat, but it is also very helpful in gaining muscles at the same time. Following it even ensures that weight relapse doesn't take place at all.

Moving on from one meal to another can get difficult if you are not having balanced meals. If you are consuming too many refined carbs, then also, you might find it difficult to move on from one meal to another without feeling the food cravings and hunger pangs.

Therefore, you must have a very balanced meal.

Managing the Macronutrients

There are 3 main components of any meal

1. Fat
2. Protein
3. Carbohydrate

You must consume all these macronutrients in a balanced manner. Having a nutrient-dense meal always helps in curbing hunger pangs for a long, and suppressing food cravings.

The ideal distribution of the macronutrients should be in the ratio given below:

Fat: 70-75% Fat is dense, and the body takes a lot of time to process fats. This means that when you consume a fat-rich diet, it keeps you feeling full for longer, and prevents hunger pangs. The body takes much longer in processing the fats, and this also helps in preventing the insulin spike in your body. You can easily get a lot of calories even by eating fat in small quantities. When you have to consume a lot of calories in fewer meals, making fat the main component of your meal always helps.

However, you must ensure that you eat healthy fats. You can get healthy fats from animal meat, fish, nuts, seeds, and fruits. 1 gram of fat provides 9 calories. It is more than double the number of calories received from carbs of the same weight. This means you can get more calories by consuming fat in smaller quantities. You must include healthy fats in your diet to stay satiated.

Protein: 20-25% Protein is essential for your muscle building. When your body is running on a low-carb diet, and you are doing a lot of exercises, there is a loss of muscle mass. The muscles are constantly breaking, and new ones are building. To help this process, you will need to consume a lot of protein. Therefore, protein should form the second biggest part of your meals.

However, you should never consume protein in excess as that would again get broken as glucose.

You can get protein from lean meats, fish, nuts, dairy, egg white, and legumes. Try to have protein in moderate amounts to ensure that you get the required protein from your meals.

Carbohydrate: 5-10% Carbohydrate should constitute the smallest part of your meal. You must not consume refined carbs as they get processed very quickly, and increase the blood sugar levels.

However, once the body processes the refined carbs, you would start feeling hungry again. Consumption of refined carbs would lead to food cravings and hunger pangs.

You must consume complex carbohydrates like whole grains that take a lot of time to get processed and give your gut a lot of fiber in the end. This not only helps in keeping your blood sugar levels low but is also very good for your gut ecosystem. Several important trace minerals are only found in whole grains, and that's why they are so important.

Green leafy vegetables are the second most important source of carbohydrates that you must consume. Green leafy vegetables do not only have a lot of fiber, but also vitamins and minerals in huge quantities. They help you with a lot of antioxidants, phytonutrients, and flavonoids that help fight chronic inflammations.

You must consume at least 7-8 cups of green leafy vegetables every day for a healthy body.

There are several benefits of consuming green leafy vegetables in large quantities. First, they are very low in calories, and hence you can consume them in any quantity you like without worrying about the calories consumed. Second, the green leafy vegetables provide a gel-like fiber to your body that helps your gut a lot. It helps in keeping your digestive system clean. You wouldn't face problems like constipation and other such issues. Third, green leafy vegetables can be consumed in large quantities, and hence they help you in feeling fuller for longer.

You can eat them as salads, or even make a smoothie as per your liking. However, it is always advisable to avoid starchy vegetables in large quantities, as they just add calories to your system and raise your blood sugar levels.

Three-Stage Process for 16/8 Intermittent Fasting Protocol

If you follow the procedure in the same order, you will face the least difficulty and discomfort. Your body will get the time to adjust to the change, and there would be no long-term side effects.

- Elimination of Snacks
- Shorter 12/12 fasting
- 16/8 intermittent fasting

Elimination of Snacks. Frequent snacking is more of a habitual issue rather than a physiological one. Most of us have become a part of modern food culture. There is food all around us. We have easy and affordable access to ready-made food that is tempting and tasty. From street food to fast-food chains, the options are unlimited. Even the audio-visual mediums like television, movies, theaters, and clubs highly promote the consumption of food. This makes eating frequently a habit. Most of the time we are not eating, because we are hungry, but because the food is lying in front of us. You are never really hungry for the pop-corns while you are watching a movie. You have been initiated into feeling that hunger. However, that has become a part of our life, and this is among the first things that you will need to change.

You cannot have snacks. You will have to learn to transition from one meal to another without having snacks. It may sound extremely difficult, but it isn't. Slight adjustments in the composition of your meals and a little bit of self-control will be more than enough to do the trick for you. If you still feel the urge to have something, you can have some of the permitted beverages like unsweetened fresh lime water, black tea, and coffee.

The first step towards the successful implementation of an intermittent fasting strategy is to eliminate all kinds of snacks from your life. You can have three meals a day. These three meals should be balanced and nutritious. You can include the food items of your choice, and you must try to remove sweets and refined carbs from these meals. Sugar-rich food items, refined carbs, aerated beverages add a lot of empty calories to your body that spikes your blood sugar levels.

However, they do not give anything substantial to your gut for processing. This confuses your body as the gut begins the digestion process, but gets nothing to process. The body uses up the glucose fuel in a short while, hence, you again start feeling the hunger pangs.

Having a balanced diet that has lots of healthy fats, proteins, and fiber gives your gut the things to process. Fiber takes up a lot of space in the gut and gets processed slow. The same happens with fat and protein. This means that your gut would remain busy for long, and hence you wouldn't feel the hunger pangs.

Having a healthy diet is a good way to get rid of the habit of frequent snacking. You must also place your meals at equal intervals as that will help in creating healthy gaps between the meals.

Shorter 12/12 Fasts. This is the easiest fasting routine to follow. You would simply need to remain in the fasted state for 12 hours, and use the remaining 12 hours for having your meals. You must use the 12 hours of your eating window to place the three meals equidistantly. Once you have gained reasonable control over your habit of snacking, it would become very easy.

Normally, we spend 7-8 hours of sleep. This is the time when you wouldn't have an urge to eat. You can have your last meal of the day 3-4 hours before bedtime, and that would do the trick. A healthy meal takes much longer than that to get processed, and hence, you wouldn't feel hunger pangs before sleeping.

We generally don't have our meals as soon as we get up, and that gives us another 2-3 hours before our first meal. This means that it will be very easy to manage 12 hours of fasting in a normal routine.

The purpose of this routine is to get out of the habit of indiscriminate eating simply. This may look like overemphasizing a simple point, but it isn't. People who have erratic sleeping patterns have a habit of eating late at night. If they don't take proper meals at night, grabbing a can of soda or munching on a pack of chips while watching TV is very common, and that can do all the damage. It will keep spiking your blood sugar levels, and insulin resistance would keep increasing.

To remain healthy and free from insulin resistance, it is important that you strictly follow the 12-hour fasting window. You must follow this routine for a considerable period before moving on to the next step. Your body must get adjusted and comfortable to this schedule before you move on to the next step.

The 16/8 Intermittent Fasting Routine. This is the real deal that you have to focus on. The 16/8 intermittent fasting routine is very easy to follow once you have got rid of the habit of snacking, and have developed the restraint to remain in the fasted state for 12 hours straight.

In this routine, you will need to remain in the fasted state for 16 hours and will get an 8-hour eating window. It is always best to begin your fasting window early in the evening and extend it as far as possible until the next day.

If you are a morning person and wake up early, you would start feeling the urge to eat soon. Therefore, you must begin your fast early in the evening. If you generally wake up between 6-7 in the morning and like to have your breakfast between 8-9, your fasting window should begin around 5 in the evening.

If you are a night person and remain awake till late, you can have the last meal of the day a bit late and extend your first meal further into the day. However, you must try to have your last meal of the day at least 3-4 hours before going to bed. This would give your body ample time to begin the digestion process. Going to bed immediately after having your meal is never a good idea. The food never gets processed properly, and you will have digestion issues.

Therefore, from a health point of view, it is important to have dinner at least 3-4 hours before hitting the bed. This also gives you the advantage that you wouldn't have to remain hungry for long once you wake up.

Remember that the urge to eat would be the strongest in the morning, and hence having dinner early in the evening helps in avoiding any kind of discomfort caused by the hunger pangs. You would be able to have food early in the day.

You will need to manage

Poor Satiety Levels. Although I may be using the word 'easy' very liberally, to a beginner, it wouldn't be very easy. Remaining hungry is never such an easy task, especially if you are already obese. I don't say this with sarcasm, but with the knowledge that obesity can lead to hormonal imbalances that will create issues with the satiety levels of the person suffering from it.

Obese people generally also suffer from chronic inflammations in fat cells. It leads to an imbalance in the release of 'leptin' the satiety hormone. This means that you may not feel satisfied even after eating the required amount of food. You may even start feeling hunger pangs in a short while after having the meals.

This happens due to leptin resistance in your body. However, this is a phenomenon that can improve once you start showing restraint on your eating habits. It may be difficult for a few days initially. However, your satiety levels would improve tremendously over some time.

Food Cravings. Food cravings remain a problem in the initial days for people who have too much sugar in their diet or eat a carbohydrate-rich diet. Sugar and refined carbs in the food lead to cravings. Simply eating something sweet doesn't solve the problem, as the more you treat yourself with sugar, the greater the urge to have it. The best way to handle food cravings is to make some positive changes in the diet. A diet rich in fat, protein, whole grains, and fiber will not only help you in feeling a greater level of satiety but will also eliminate the problem of frequent food cravings.

Headaches. A nagging headache can be a problem for people starting intermittent fasting or making a change in their diet. Once you start having a high-fat low-carb diet and lower the consumption of sugar and refined carbs, your body starts struggling to find the sugar. You will have sugar withdrawal symptoms, and the headache is one of those symptoms.

The good thing is that, if you start getting headaches, it means your body has started the transition. It indicates that you are on the right path, and your body will start experiencing fat-burning soon.

To manage the headaches, you can simply take the help of unsweetened black tea or coffee. These beverages help in dealing with these headaches that may trouble you in the beginning.

Lightheadedness. This is another problem that almost everyone faces when beginning intermittent fasting. You can feel:

1. Your legs shaky while walking
2. Momentary darkness before your eyes when you stand up from a squatting position
3. Difficulty in maintaining balance when you stand up very quickly
4. Difficulty in concentration
5. Problems in focusing on any particular thing

All these are symptoms of sugar withdrawal, and they are Temporary. These symptoms will go away within a couple of days.

These things happen because your body craves sugar supply. It stops getting glucose from food at regular intervals, and it creates these symptoms as a part of its protest. However, within a few days, the body switches to burning fat for fuel, and because it is a more reliable, long-lasting, and cleaner medium of energy that even creates lower waste and toxins, these symptoms go away.

Thoughts of Ditching the Routine. Our body has a very sophisticated fight or flight response for everything. Whenever we get into any sort of crisis, the mind creates the fight or flight response in which it tries to find the easiest way to get out of the problem. Fighting hunger is never a lucrative idea for your brain, as it may create an energy crisis. It would try to lure you into ditching the routine. It happens with every weight loss regimen. You would feel more tempted to eat things that you didn't even like in particular. Your mind would keep thinking about food all the time.

You may start feeling tired, weak, and depressed. These are all feelings created to motivate you towards ditching the routine. If you want to lose weight and lead a healthy life, you will have to face them bravely and strongly for a few days as they pass away very soon.

Chapter 4

Suitable people to go for Intermittent Fasting 16/8

With fasting, comes a lot of patience and gratitude towards the importance of food and with time, our stamina to go without food for extended periods builds up. Our eating habits change, and with the benefits of IF 16/8, we can turntables.

Without any doubt, IF 16/8 is trending for the right reasons, but does it have the same effects for both men and women? From internal body functions to looks, to odors, everything varies between both the sexes. Is it the same for both genders in the case of intermittent fasting?

It's sad to hear, but it does not affect men and women the same way since in terms of weight loss it is more efficient in men. Men can fast for a longer period without any side effects; however, in women, it can be problematic if not done the right way. Well, there is no answer to why every person's anatomy is different, and when considering genders, they are very unique.

A girl has to go through her menstrual cycle as soon as she enters her teenage, and from there starts the hormonal changes as the body starts growing. For girls, the production of estrogen and progesterone results in the growth of your breasts and the development of the uterus and fallopian tubes.

A girl changes to a woman as the body makes the areas around the waist and hips more prominent, with more facial hair growth as well as hair growth on the arms, legs, and vagina.

When a girl gets married, she has to go through her pregnancy periods bearing a child in her womb. With all these body evolution procedures, changes in the hormone level can harm the women.

For men, puberty starts a little late in teens than in women. The development of the body to manhood starts with the production of the hormone, testosterone. This male sex hormone is responsible for sperm production in men. A boy's chest widens, and hair growth on the body begins.

With all these functioning and energy-requiring processes going on in the body, staying without food can affect the body negatively, especially for women. Because hormones are and have been altered by our diet, we need to make sure that gender differences are kept in mind.

Since the time of the hunter-gatherers, women have played their roles as wives, mothers, and helpers as their men went on to hunt food. At that time, bearing children was a necessary tradition to increase the number of helping hands and to continue their legacy. It took time to find a meal.

To reproduce, do chores and bear with their menstrual cycle, women needed energy, and therefore their lifestyles affected their body development. Not only did these ancestral women require building their muscles and store fats, but they also had to sustain them to carry out their biological functions. Thus, historically it makes sense that fasting and hormones have a connection.

According to research in collaboration with the Department of Nuclear Medicine and the Royal Sussex Hospital, unlike men, women are less glucose tolerant.

They have less amount of hepatic extraction of insulin and also breakdown less glycogen to glucose when exercising. This proves that men have to work out lesser than women to lose the same amount of fat, and therefore, they should take no pride as they flaunt their muscular bodies.

With these clear differences in genders, the different responses of the body towards intermittent fasting are pretty obvious. In men, IMF can work as well as up to 99 percent, while for women the weight loss is mainly due to muscle reduction, which contributes to 25 percent of the weight loss. This is not healthy, as women and any normal human being need to sustain muscle. In men, intermittent fasting can boost levels of testosterone in reliance on glucose concentration. As the insulin levels are more actively triggered during the day, men can skip the morning breakfast.

This way it also increases the metabolic functioning in men and makes them more active during the day. Ultimately, it responds with a decrease in leptin which increases the testosterone levels.

Looking at fasting in general, it might decrease testosterone levels, but intermittent fasting works in its ways.

As mentioned in the above chapters, this diet plan was initially performed by bodybuilders, and therefore can also result in significant changes in athletes. What do you think? Will the overall positive impact of intermittent fasting have the same impact on athletes? Athletes aim to maintain their optimal body weight, and research proved it to be accomplishable.

34 athletes in an 8-week study along with endurance training were to undergo intermittent fasting, the time-restricted feeding way.

These athletes consumed their nutrient-dense meals in the 8-hour duration only, and thus they had lost weight with negligible muscle loss along with no enhanced physical performance. These athletes felt better within themselves.

There was a great loss in adipose tissue mass. IMF 16/8 or time-restricted feeding, when compared to a 3 day fast, has a negative anaerobic capacity control.

Ketones are released into the bloodstream when fats are burned to release energy. Ketones have the power to reduce weight and offer security by saving some brain functions. They provide security against Alzheimer's disease, a memory loss disorder in which slowly and steadily your memory starts fading and then is lost completely. A study included 23 elderly people with impairments who were subject to either a very high or a deficient carbohydrate diet for six weeks. A moderate correlation of insulin with memory was found out, with no relationship to weight.

The study proved memory gain in all 23 adults, and further research also discovered that intermittent fasting promotes healthy and normal growth of nerve cells in the brain thus making the nerve signals more efficient and active.

Preserving your muscle mass is the best thing you can do to your body because even at rest it makes you burn calories. This is the consequence of intermittent fasting. Clinical researches on male mice showed that there were muscle mass increases and an overall decrease in insulin levels. These mice were kept under observation for 8 weeks. Half of them were fed with a high-fat diet and the other half with a low-fat diet.

Our young generation has been a target of deep depression and anxiety issues as they deal with increased stress in their lives. This disrupts their lifestyles with late-night snacks and an upside-down sleeping routine. Intermittent fasting is a solution for improved psychological well-being and mental stress. It also reduces chronic inflammation, which can be a factor leading to added weight gain and health-related problems. With all these benefits, it increases the estimated lifespan of an individual. At least in rats, the lifespan has increased by 33% to 83%.

Remember that be it, men or women, both need to adapt to healthy diets along with correctly set lifestyles to let the magic of intermittent fasting begin. Both of them should take nutrient-rich food during their feeding window, as they are on calorie restriction for the rest of the day. Men do well in lifestyle adjustments than women, so what are women supposed to do?

How exactly does intermittent fasting affect the menstrual cycle and cause hormonal imbalance? Should they not practice intermittent fasting 16/8 and if they do, what precautions are they supposed to take? Is it even effective for women? How can women keep their biological functions in control along with intermittent fasting? We will cover all these questions in further subchapters, so continue reading to know more.

Moreover, let's not stick to fasting in terms of weight loss only, as research in animals and humans during the last century has opened health-related feedbacks regarding intermittent fasting which includes hormonal balancing, keto-genesis, decreasing oxidative tension, burning, inflammation, and increased stress resistance and lipolysis.

Human clinical research also points out that fasting improves hypertension, joint pain, heart disease, metabolic syndrome, osteoarthritis, and improved quality of life.

Intermittent Fasting for Women

You must be thinking that women should choose some other diet plan as even after putting in the same effort as men, they are not benefiting with the same result.

Well, although it sounds like this, it is not. Let's not rush to conclusions and discuss all the points one by one in detail. The luteinizing hormone is responsible for the menstrual and egg cycle in the ovaries of a woman, while the hormone testosterone balances the reproductive system in men. When a woman starts her intermittent fasting routine, she cuts down on extra calories and eats only for limited periods.

As soon as her body calorie meter drops below a specific level, the woman enters a low energy level zone with high stress, and the hormones are unfavorably affected.

Along with all the body changes occurring in a body, this puts an unexpected break to the menstrual cycle causing fertility problems. The fatigue, the diet plan makes men and women face is severe for the latter.

Missing periods is not at all healthy, and it means that not only your sex hormones but all the other hormones are disturbed as well. No one knows why women are so sensitive to IF, but studies even in female rats prove that it provokes the reproductive system.

According to a study for intermittent fasting of about 3 to 6 months on female rats, the ovaries shrank and the rats ended up with a disturbed menstrual cycle. The solution to this is to carry on the fasting routine but with shorter fasting durations and fewer days.

This moderate approach will not starve women, neither will it send signals to the hypothalamus nor will there be any chances of a reproductive shutdown occurring. They will also get a longer eating window and hunger pangs leading to a slow and gradual adaptation to the fasting period.

A 14/10 hours window is best considered for women. The fetus and mother relationship is only a "take" relation where the fetus takes all the nutrients it requires and even dilates the blood vessels surrounding it according to its need and comfort.

This increases the mother's appetite, and so this type of fasting is not recommended during pregnancy, or else it could be harmful to both the child and parent. The main reason why women face all these difficulties compared to men is scientifically embedded in their genes; the hormones in a woman's body are programmed to prevent her fetus from starving, even when she's not pregnant, so a woman is overall very sensitive to anything that resembles a starvation signal.

Therefore, scientists relate it to the relationship between a virus and its host. The virus enters the host, takes all its needs in the form of nutrients to replicate, and then starts living inside the host as if it has been a living organism since the beginning. While some women might face these issues, others have no negative effects. It once again shows how different we all are. It's not like intermittent fasting is not effective in women. It can be extremely effective as long as it is done under the guidance of a specialist and dealt with care. Beyoncé herself shared that she lost 20 pounds with fasting, but she also mentioned that as soon as you get back on your normal or even low-calorie intake, you put on some of the weight you lost.

If your mind is still stuck on how long it will take for a woman to trim her waistline, you are in the wrong direction. As mentioned before, women just need to adopt a healthy lifestyle and change the fasting window according to their suitability.

They must keep a check with their fitness trainers and doctors. Obviously, with time, intermittent fasting will eventually help them lose that fat, but it should not be at the expense of their health.

There are also some less extreme variants of IF though, where you need simply to miss a meal. Try this version and see how your body responds. This relaxed approach is called the crescendo method of intermittent fasting. The idea behind it is to not mess up your hormones with a shock.

A review of six studies on intermittent fasting was performed in 2018 over 3 to 12 months, which concluded that the weight loss consists of an average of 15 pounds.

Another case study from participants that went through a shorter 3 to 24-week research program also showed that the reduction in inches was approximately 7%, which is a positive result.

Coming to health, fasting improves it. Be it a woman or a man, intermittent fasting helps you get rid of diabetes and heart diseases. A study on 16 obese men and women experimented with alternate-day fasting for 10 weeks with three phases.

During the controlled food intake and 2 weeks of selected food intake, the weight loss remained constant. After 8 weeks, there was a drop in body fat of about 3%. More importantly, the systolic blood pressure changed from 124 to 116 mm Hg with a tremendous change in the cholesterol level. It showed how the triglycerides lowered by 32% and cholesterol by 25%. This clearly shows favorable results of intermittent fasting in terms of heart health even when the fast is 24 hours long one with no food, where fluids are allowed, but they should be calorie-free.

Diabetic patients have a high blood sugar level, and therefore, either their bodies do not make enough insulin or are not using the available insulin properly. In these cases, they differentiate as type-1 and type-2 diabetes.

This keeps your blood concentrated and can result in various problems like cardiovascular diseases, respiratory issues, and even conceiving can be difficult with fewer chances of ovulation. According to numerous studies, intermittent fasting may reduce the probability of having diabetes, and for pre-diabetic patients, it can lessen the risks.

107 overweight pre-menopausal women were tested with intermittent fasting for over 6 months. The blood sugar remained consistent. It lowered insulin levels by almost 29% so that the glucose concentration in the blood would not increase any further.

A similar study of intermittent fasting of 8 to 12 weeks not only decreased the insulin levels but also lowered the blood glucose concentration by up to 6% in pre-diabetic individuals. These were the ones with high blood sugar levels but were not diabetic.

In addition to this, it also releases oxidative stress and decreases the inflammation process in women. It keeps the cell stress response more alert and provides a woman with more energy than during the normal routine.

However, if you experience any of the following symptoms, it should be discontinued immediately: extreme hair fall, sleeping disorders such as insomnia, bad dreams, menstrual irregularities, acne or rashes, uncontrollable stress, and anxiety attacks, mood swings, reduced libido, slowed digestion and constant shivering. All of this can also generate negative energy balance which makes the body weak. The signals are not able to figure out the difference between a real and an imaginary threat to the body. On the other hand, both the crescendo and lean gains fasting methods of intermittent fasting are safe for women.

IF gives mental and physical benefits which makes it all the more fun to do, but women should design this plan keeping some tips into consideration. Coming on to what they exactly mean by a relaxed or moderate approach?

- First of all, as a beginner decide your fasting and feeding time frames and periods. It is better if you approach a 14 to 10-hour window as a woman, but even if you are experienced, do not fast for longer than 24 hours. If you do fast for 24 hours, keep them to a minimum of 2 fasts per week. The ideal window would be 12 to 16 hours.
- Do not reach the consistency of fasting for 7 days regularly as a starter up till the next 3 weeks minimum at least.
- Drink plenty of water, herbal tea, bone broth, and low-calorie fluids.
- Have high-density meals during your eating window.
- Keep your exercise routine light on fasting days like gentle stretching, walking, and yoga, etc. Avoid doing cardio and weight lifting workouts.

16/8 Intermittent Fasting for Men

The 16/8 intermittent fasting protocol for men is among the most successful and widely followed ways to lose weight and gain good health.

You can divide your day into 2 parts:

- The Fasting Window

- The Eating Window

The best thing about 16/8 intermittent fasting is that it can be made a part of your daily life. It doesn’t ask you to do anything extra, and hence, it is easy to follow. There are only two things to be kept in mind.

- The hours within which you can eat
- The things you should eat

The success of any weight loss plan depends on your dedication to that plan, and intermittent fasting is no exception. Although intermittent fasting puts no holds on the things you can eat and the things you can’t. Yet, it is expected of you to show a reasonable attitude towards food items.

- You shouldn't eat unhealthy things
- You can't eat things in excess quantities
- You mustn't eat outside your eating window

The Fasting Window. The fasting window should generally begin early in the evening when you are about to finish the active part of the day. There are several benefits to beginning the fasting window at the end of the day.

- You’d get in the resting mode
- Your chances of getting invited to eat something by friends and colleagues would get low
- You’d be in a more relaxed atmosphere
- Your body would get at least 3-4 hours to digest the food before you hit the bed. Your gut would be grateful for that

Ideally, the fasting window should begin anywhere between 5-7 in the evening. Men should fast for at least 16 hours, which means if you begin your fast around 5 in the evening, you will be able to have the first meal of the day around 9.

If you take it at 7 in the evening, the first meal would not be possible before 11 in the day. Pushing it any further can keep pushing the first meal of the day farther into the day.

This may not look like a big issue at the moment, but believe me; it's something you should worry about. It takes around 4-5 hours before your gut can properly process a healthy meal; therefore, it is very unlikely that you would feel any hunger pang before hitting the bed. However, things would be different when you wake up.

Even if you sleep for 7-8 hours, the total fasting time would have been around 12 hours when you wake up. This is the time the hunger starts to build up. If you maintain a healthy exercise routine, you wouldn't feel very hungry for another 1-2 hours as physical activity suppresses the feeling of hunger momentarily.

However, the hunger would start building up pretty strongly after that. I am assuming that you would also need to go to work. Passing the next one or two hours in the fasted state while working can be difficult. Therefore, it is always best to begin the fasting window early, so that you can get the first meal of the day before you start the active part of the day.

- Begin your fasting window as early as possible, and try to make it a routine.
- Don't shift the timings a lot as your body would also need to adjust to the routine
- It is important that you somewhat fix the timings of your first and last meal of the day

Eating Window. You get 8 hours for the eating window. These 8 hours are important as you will need to take all the nutrition during these 8 hours. It may look like a lot of time, but it isn't.

After 16 hours of fasting, when you have the first meal of the day, it is generally very difficult to have another meal after 4 hours. You will also need to ensure that you don't indulge in overeating.

If you don't have a properly balanced meal, transitioning from one meal to another smoothly without the urge to have something in between will become difficult.

Therefore, you must have a very balanced first meal of the day. It should have all the macronutrients and should provide the required minerals and vitamins that your body needs.

The first meal of the day is important as it is going to be the most fulfilling meal for you. It is always best that you get it at home. You get complete control over the ingredients of your meal, and the way you prepare it. If you have your meals out, you can't be sure of these things.

You must always remember that food is a very important part of any weight-loss strategy, therefore, you can't ignore this part completely. Although you can have 3 meals in the 8 hours eating window, it is generally not possible to have 3 proper meals in this short gap. If you have a healthy and fulfilling meal at the start of the day, you are not likely to have the urge to have a complete meal at lunch.

The lunch should be light as it can make you feel lethargic. Generally, the last meal of the day is the second proper meal you will be able to have, and that's why you will have to focus on the first and last meal.

Exercise. Exercise is another important part of an intermittent fasting routine. Intermittent fasting helps your body in getting into fat-burning mode.

However, it is your job to create the energy demand. If you are leading a highly active life, then that can come naturally, but the chances of the same are slim. This makes it important that you create the energy demands through exercise.

High-Intensity Interval Training is one of the best ways to create high energy demands quickly. It pushes your body to burn calories faster. Intermittent fasting also leads to an increase in the production of HGH in your body, and that also helps in increasing your fat-burning abilities through exercise.

- You will need to remain in the fasted state for at least 16 hours in a day to get the maximum benefits.
- The longer you would fast, the better the results would be.
- You should try to extend the fasting hours as much as possible.
- The best strategy to do so would be to begin the fasting early and start pushing the breakfast later into the day.
- You should reduce the intake of refined carbs and sugar in your diet.
- You should also reduce your reliance on processed food items as much as possible.
- The shift towards the whole and unprocessed food items.
- Drink plenty of fluids.
- You can have unsweetened black tea and coffee, and even fresh lime water for suppressing the hunger pangs.
- However, you should avoid excessive consumption of tea or coffee in both the fasting as well as eating windows.
- You must take as much rest as possible.
- Sleeping for at least 7-8 hours is very important for faster weight loss.

Chapter 5

Intermittent Fasting and your metabolism

There are two major explanations for intermittent fasting success.

They are periods of short fasting followed by periods of normal calorie intake.

- This fasting method is that extremely low or no-calorie consumption is only done for short periods. A continued fast without returning to normal calorie intake will slow down the body's metabolism. However, short periods of fasting, like the 5:2 or 16:8 method appear to maintain and possibly increase your body burning calories.
  Then continuous fluctuation of fasting and normal food consumption keeps your body on its toes, rather than allowing the metabolism to slow down.
- Do not compare normal calorie intake to binging or excessive eating. What normal intake means is taking in what the body's approximate calorie needs is by eating a variety of healthy foods. It doesn't mean eating or binging on favorite foods that are unhealthy and have empty calories.

You may, after completing a fasting day, determined to continue consuming very low calories. This concept is very simple and you will know more later.

To keep the metabolism stoked and continue burning fat, your body needs a day of consuming a normal number of calories.

If you continue to maintain extremely low-calorie intake day after day without a break, your metabolism will slow down because the body will eventually go into starvation mode.

However, when done properly, intermittent fasting seems to be reasonably safe and could be a better and more effective manner to diet, as well as improving your health.

1 - Fasting and the brain

Creates more brain cells. Fasting increases the rates of neurogenesis, which is the growth and development of new brain cells and nerve tissues, in the brain. Brain performance, focus, mood, and memory are connected to higher rates of neurogenesis. (Salcido, Dr. Brady, 2017)

Increases BDNF in the Brain. Fasting not only increases your rate of neurogenesis, but it also increases the production of BDNF, an important protein that has played a role in neuroplasticity and allows the brain to continue to adapt and change.

The brain is much stronger, adaptable to change, and more resilient to stress.

The BDNF gene gives instructions for making a protein produced inside nerve cells. It produces new brain cells that protect your brain cells and stimulates new synapses and connections while increasing memory, learning, and improves moods.

Reduces Inflammation (Salcido, Dr. Brady, 2017). Intermittent fasting reduces inflammation. There are many ways of intermittent fasting to reduce inflammation.

- Insulin Sensitivity – Fasting shows that it helps solve insulin resistance. Insulin and glucose build up in the blood and create inflammation when the body becomes resistant to insulin. Intermittent fasting gives the body a break. With no food to digest and the sugar stores are used up by the body, insulin levels begin to drop and lets the body re-sensitize to insulin again.
- Ketones – While fasting, all the sugar stores are used by the body and have to turn to the fat stores for fuel. Ketones are created when fat is broken down. The ketones that are responsible for regulating inflammatory diseases like

arthritis and Alzheimer's are B-hydroxybutyrate that blocks part of the immune system.

- Autophagy – stimulates autophagy so the body cleanses itself and reduces inflammation.

2 - Burns fat for fuel

Surprisingly, fat is a cleaner and effective source of fuel rather than carbohydrates. Fat not only produces more energy per gram than carbohydrates do, but it can produce fewer free radicals, the cause of inflammation.

When fat (ketones) or carbohydrates are used by your mitochondria, your cell batteries to make energy, there is a waste that gets produced which are free radicals.

The body goes through oxidative stress caused by free radicals and is thought to be the cause of chronic diseases, including neurodegenerative diseases.

3 - Boosts your energy

Intermittent fasting has been linked with the increase of mitochondrial biogenesis, the creation of new mitochondria. As previously mentioned, mitochondria are the batteries for your cells. Mitochondria fill each cell and power the cells to do their job.

The cells' job is to take the food you eat and change it into energy. The brain gains more brainpower when you have mitochondria in the brain.

4 - Boosts HIGH Levels

HGH levels are naturally increased to give health, anti-aging, repair, longevity, and neuroprotective benefits by intermittent fasting. HGH can give neuroprotection, improve cognition, and increase neurogenesis.

Muscle mass and Intermittent Fasting

Fat mass and lean mass, which is everything besides fat, including muscle, will be lost when there is a loss of weight, and no exercise is included in a diet program. This is true of weight loss caused by both conventional diets and intermittent fasting.

Gaining muscle during intermittent fasting is another story. Research is very limited as to whether it is possible to do so or not. This is probably because weight loss is the topic in most studies about these diets.

A study was conducted where a group of men were on a conventional diet or time-restricted eating program and completed a weight training program over eight weeks.

Before the study, the group had not previously performed any weight training regularly. During the study, the group was expected to eat all their food in a four-hour time frame, four days a week.

At the end of the study, the men who were in the time-restricted eating group maintained lean body mass, and their strength increased. The other group who followed the conventional diet gained five pounds of lean mass and also increased their strength.

The study showed that intermittent fasting is not best for muscle gain. It is possible that the time-restricted eating group ate less protein than the conventional diet group.

Other scientifically-based reasons are why intermittent fasting may not be ideal for gaining muscle. You need to eat more calories than you burn to gain muscle, consume enough protein so that your body can build new muscle tissue, and have adequate exercise inducement to cause growth.

Additionally, to get enough protein, you may have to make a greater effort when eating less often than with a conventional diet.

All the reasons given do not mean that gaining muscle is impossible when following intermittent fasting, but it may not be easy to gain muscle.

It is highly recommended that exercise, such as weight training while intermittent fasting helps in maintaining muscle, even when you lose fat. Additionally, other forms of exercise such as elliptical or a stationary bike may benefit maintaining muscle.

Chapter 6

Strategies for losing weight quickly

Some strategies make your life easier by reaching your target of weight loss quickly. It's important to look healthy and happy with a thinner body. These strategies are to be noted and memorized at your fingertips. The two main strategies that have a huge contribution to weight loss are increasing your fasting window and having a high-calorie deficit. All the other tips will be summarized along with the main points.

Increasing your fasting window will lead to weight loss, but not with the powerful biological effects of intermittent fasting.

At the initial stage, start your fast after dinner so that it passes as you sleep and also improves your adherence to dieting. Keep your window short to around 12 hours, especially if you are a woman.

Stick to a routine by setting up one. Start and break your fast at regular timings every day. The routine will also keep you away from boredom. It's tough to manage time when you have work, family life, and other life circumstances, but here we have the benefit.

One way is to slowly increase your fasting window to 16 hours. The other way is to keep changing the timings every day according to routine. These alterations have been mentioned before in detail.

The third way is to fast for the number of hours you desire every day, following your hectic working hours, starting from 12 hours onwards. This way you can adapt to many routines and set the plan for your entire week. Set day one with a fasting period of 14 hours, day two with 12 hours, day three with 18 hours, and so on.

When you have the will, you can find the way and get that chic body you have to give in your best. If you cannot handle it, get yourself a dose of caffeine early morning and in the afternoon.

The 16/8 method is famous for being similar to the normal routine with no difficult challenges as such.

HELENA is to date, the most extensive research done on Intermittent Fasting. The German Cancer Hospital was also involved in the process but is not in favor of the diet routine in the long run. 150 obese individuals were examined for the study and divided accordingly into three groups.

The first group followed a calorie restriction method that reduced the calorie intake by about 20% through the 16/8 protocol. The second group was supposed to follow the 5:2 plan or alternate fasting routine. The third group being the control group just had to take a balanced diet.

This process was then continued for the next 38 weeks. The purpose of the study was to find out whether intermittent fasting is a healthy way of reducing weight. The results turned out to be surprising.

Both methods proved to be equal in terms of health and weight loss effects. The belly fat was reduced too. Some people may find it easy to control themselves within 2 days only instead of a whole week adjustment. It is better to switch to a balanced diet anyhow.

Kuhn, the leading scientist of the research thinks that it is best to choose a dietary method and keep consistency. He says that the health effects will be achieved any way from the weight loss so why not choose something that benefits the lifestyle. Having a high-calorie deficit will directly lead you to weight loss.

Weight loss by the loss of excess body fat is completely healthy and also releases greater energy during its breakdown. This keeps the dopamine, a neurotransmitter, satisfied as it is responsible for the control of emotions.

It's critical to have micro and macronutrients added to your diet, but a high-calorie diet will spoil it all. Although you have the leverage of eating bread, rice, pizza, pasta, etc. it is always beneficial and effective to approach the protein-rich diet. These high carbohydrates food items not only raise your blood sugar, blood pressure, and fat, but also cause extreme mood swings and depression. This does not mean you cannot have any carbohydrates or fat. It just reminds you to have healthier options.

For intermittent fasting, this can be beef, fish, fruits, veggies, avocados, and almonds. Nuts are healthy fats that provide a lot of calories with just a small portion, and therefore their intake should be kept in minimal quantities. Soups are a convenient option for a meal replacement as they provide lesser calories than solid foods and are satiating too.

Other power tips include keeping yourself hydrated enough to lower your appetite and for the body to perform its functions. The water intake gives your stomach the perception of being full, which signals the brain regarding the feeling.

Green tea can also make the experience way easier than it is by suppressing and curbing your hunger pangs. The overall process shall increase your body's metabolic efficiency. During your fed state, it is tough to manage fat burning as your insulin levels are increasing, so the only duration that gives you a chance for fat burning is your fasting state.

After your last meal, the body enters the post-absorptive state where the body has a low insulin level and is not ready to further process any more meals. Having more meals and snacks will raise insulin levels and instead of breaking down, it will be stored as fats.

Eat carefully as your body will always prefer burning sugars before any other source.

Therefore, no carbohydrates should be eaten. Without any readily available glucose or glycogen units, your body will have no choice, but to force the fat cells to breakdown for energy. Post-workout, the glucose in your muscles has already been depleted as the aerobic and anaerobic respiration used it, but the meal we will be consuming now will either be stored to replace the burned glycogen in the muscles or will be broken straight away. Therefore, post-workout meals even if they are high in calories are always good to have.

Let's just switch to lettuce and broccoli as our favorites rather than Margherita pizzas with pepperoni. Thus, the strategies conclude that when you do eat, it should be with mindfulness and moderation while overdoing nothing (including fat). Get your 8 hours of sleep and feel rested. Do not over exhaust yourself.

After having gone through 40 studies review by the Harvard Chan School of Health, it was found that intermittent fasting was an efficient measure for weight loss. Individuals would lose within 7lbs to 11lbs over 2.5 months. They have also figured out how the locking of the mitochondria in one state can block the effects of intermittent fasting.

To maintain weight with Intermittent Fasting 16/8

In 2016, the World Health Organization reported that more than 1.9 billion people were overweight and over 650 million people were obese in the world. With obesity comes a lot of diseases and risk factors towards one's life and most individuals tend to lose their self-confidence.

The more they are shattered watching themselves in an extra-large outfit, the more motivation they get to lose weight. As intermittent fasting is the king of diet routines currently, it not only helps shed the extra pounds but also guides the way to maintain the weight once the target is achieved.

A review of all the four studies by Davis et al. proves that intermittent fasting and other dietary plans had great weight loss in intermittent fasting groups. Seimon et al. in their review figured that short and long-term interventions are both suitable for intermittent fasting as well as calorie restriction diet plans, but the calorie restriction causes hunger and binge eating as the calorie intake is very low, and becomes unbearable.

Therefore, IF is more useful in the long run, but how are we supposed to maintain the weight we achieved?

Many who followed IF 16/8 point out that as soon as they left the routine and came back to their normal eating pattern, they gained some of the weight back. Is it true? What is the point of controlling yourself so long if it acts only till you live it? To practice, the 16/8 protocol might not be as tough as maintaining it.

At the end of the day, you want to smile with pride when you see yourself in the mirror. The hard work will reflect for sure, but maintaining this image is the real challenge. Being athletes or military trainees, physical activity is extremely significant. A study from the Institute of Medicine Sub-committee shows how a 10-minute exercise regime is way less effective than a 30 minute one.

Strength training with aerobics can be really helpful in weight loss, but obviously, this alone is not enough. Self-monitoring and keeping a record of your food intake and workouts in a food diary might seem old-fashioned, but to date is the most effective way of accomplishing your goal.

Carry lunch boxes with you for lunch breaks at the office and avoid fast food. Quit smoking and alcohol consumption and focus more on staying fit and healthy.

The struggle does not end with the weight loss goal being achieved. Weight maintenance has to be achieved by lifestyle changes. The determinants of body weight react to energy restriction.

A key point here is the resting energy that lowers as obese people lose weight and has been justified by experiments in both rodents and humans. Although the reduction in resting energy is dependent on body composition and size, it has been found that this energy level decreases by an unexpected amount, and therefore weight maintenance becomes an issue.

Longo's alternate-day fasting dropouts are the highest, at about 40%. This is because fasting all day can be exhausting, and therefore maintenance can be a greater issue. It can be hard to follow. Thus, this is what makes intermittent fasting 16/8 better than all the other methods.

It gives you space, and this is important. Weight maintenance can be taken care of by eating healthy and nutrient-rich food instead of junk food.

Stick to eating 3 meals in a day and no more. The energy restriction in intermittent fasting shaped the methods of intermittent fasting in weight management. However, the rebound situation is that this energy restriction scheme could result in over-consumption of energy on days that are restricted.

Food records from individuals who participated in the studies were taken. Study 1 involved around 44 women on intermittent energy restriction for 6 months, while study 2 had 4 months duration on two types of intermittent energy restriction involving 72 women.

The before and after energy intake was measured daily on restricted as well as unrestricted days and hours. By now, we all know how the consistency of days and time frames are chosen to play an important role in weight loss planning and how it affects weight loss, if it does, was recorded.

According to reports of the two studies, the intake was 21% and 29% lower than what their daily intake had been. The number of days of restriction per week was 70% for women in study 1 and 72% for women in study 2.

The group that had been consistent in their energy restriction days had lost a combined percentage weight of 6.7% to 4.7% in 3 months, while the other group had lost up to 8.7% which shows that consistency of restricted days is not linked to the success of weight loss. The main focus of the study showed that the iso-energetic diet along with the sudden reduction in the energy intake going below the baseline or the average daily intake leads to the success factors of the intermittent energy restriction fasting plan.

Despite the success of intermittent energy restriction plans in weight loss, the supporting evidence is very limited. If we did not mention it before, intermittent energy restriction could be applied to all kinds of methods such as time-restricted feeding and alternate-day fasting.

This study has examined this energy restriction program's effectiveness on overweight and obese adults in comparison to no treatment or other treatments.

Adults greater than 18 years of age were included in this study. Intermittent energy restriction was meant to consume less than 800 kilocalories on a minimum of one day per week, but a maximum of 6 days weekly. This research was extended to about 12 weeks which included post outcome results so that the review could be as accurate as possible.

This meta-analysis was completely randomized. The primary and foremost important result of this trial was in terms of change in body weight.

The second outcome would be related to the body mass index, fat mass, and waist measurements. The other categories of this outcome were health-related, such as cardiac issues, blood insulin, and glucose profiles, and blood pressure. The outcome was the shaping of their lifestyles such as nutritional guidelines and physical activity while comparing the before and after-effects.

Data was measured, and the research was continued for meta-analysis with weighted mean calculations and their 95% confidence intervals in case of any error. A total of six studies shaped the review of this research. The duration and consistency of the studies varied from 3 to 12 months and 16/8 protocols to 24 hours fast to alternate-day fasting. 4 of the studies supported the energy restriction plan, and 2 of the studies included a no-treatment control method.

The meta-analysis came in favor of intermittent fasting for weight loss than the no treatment control trial. However, intermittent energy restriction had very similar effects on continuous energy restriction for weight loss in the short run.

This confirmed that intermittent fasting is beneficial as compared to a no-treatment procedure. It should always be kept in mind to keep your lifestyle active and healthy for a happy, long life. The findings of this review have been very helpful as supporting evidence confirms that intermittent fasting has its pros that outweigh the few disadvantages it has.

How have we defined obesity or a person being overweight? Any individual with a body mass index equal to or greater than 25 and 30 makes the individual be called obese. Obesity does not only give a person complex and feelings of jealousy but causes other health issues such as chronic diseases, cancers, skeletal disorders, diabetes, etc. The Study tells that in England, the cost of treating these overweight, obese individuals is over 5 billion pounds.

Therefore, weight maintenance is mandatory for everyone throughout the world; otherwise, the economy bears the healthcare costs. The study says that doing weight management effectively can be challenging, that too when the probability of weight regains or poor long-run results can be high. It suggests that it's good to review all kinds of weight management programs to better understand their significance. Intermittent fasting protocol is a dietary approach that restricts energy intake through controlled diets and workout training for weight management.

Although the evidence has been limited, there is a way to reveal the benefits of the diet routine. This can be done by explaining the processes of fat utilization and nutritional stress.

The National Institute for Health and Care Excellence suggests not using deficient carbohydrate diets, that too as a daily intake for the treatment of obesity in adults. They suggest that this approach should be recommended only if there is a requirement for rapid weight loss. A case where pregnancy is not occurring due to extreme weight gain in an overweight individual.

In this case, too, it should be made sure that nutritional guidelines are followed and the time duration for practicing it should be a maximum of 12 weeks, that too continuously or intermittently.

Essentially, intermittent fasting uses the intermittent way of involving a very low carbohydrate diet which has also captured the attention of media. This study review was mainly to focus on wider aspects of this intervention not specifically weight loss but also looking at other benefits.

Another reason for the weight gain after or along with the weight loss is the added weight of the muscle buildup. We know that IF helps us build muscle with a natural and steady tendency.

This keeps us strong internally and externally. It also decreases our appetite and thus helps in weight sustenance through intermittent fasting 16/8.

Athletes do prefer using the intermittent fasting technique quite often along with the energy restriction to prevent any weight gain in longer periods. This population takes low energy intake daily to maintain weight, but they have to manage their workouts accordingly. Intense weight lifting training along with low energy intake will burden the athletes, cause fatigue, anaerobic respiration, irritability, and lack of performance due to low muscular strength and reflexes. In such sports, the failure to meet body conditions can result in athletes switching to even more rapid weight loss strategies that make them suffer from dehydration, palpitation, extreme sweating, and other dangerous symptoms.

Benefits of exercise

Whenever we can burn more calories than we consume, not only will we be losing weight, but we will be lowering our body fat composition. Hello, six-pack! Fasting is one of the best ways to keep our calorie intake low, but the best way to supercharge this and get the full range of benefits is by combining it with an exercise program.

First, for adults (ages 19-64) we are given a choice to some extent – whichever route you take, there should be a couple of sessions per week to work on strength exercises to keep your muscles in shape. This is going to very much complement an intermittent fasting routine since we know that will improve our lean body mass. On top of that should be either two and a half hours of moderate aerobic activity (which includes exercise such as cycling or walking briskly) per week or half that amount of time in vigorous exercise. Jogging fits this category as does, for the more competitively minded, a game of singles tennis.

That minimum activity will help maintain your weight if your calorie intake is about average. It will also support our bodies as we seek to improve heart health, organ well-being, and so on. So, for those of us fasting, this will mean weight loss-because our calorie intake will be lower than average.

So, a brisk walk at weekends and every other day during the week is going to help us lose weight. That is not a huge commitment. Two forty-minute trips to the gym will offer us the same benefits. However, there is one small caveat to this.

While such exercise regimes as mentioned above will ensure we meet our minimum targets for good health, some daily activity is also necessary. This does not have to be severe and can be broken down into ten-minute chunks. A bit of time gardening, housework – vigorous vacuuming we might say – walking the children to school – all of these will ensure we keep sufficiently on the move.

Let us take a moment to examine the health benefits of even that minimum amount of exercise. Our chances of developing type 2 diabetes are cut in half and cut the chances of heart disease or suffering a stroke by over a third.

We are more likely to live longer and some studies indicate we may reduce our chances of getting cancer by up to a half.

Our bones and muscles will serve us better and for longer. Mentally, we cut our risk of depression and of getting dementia by a third. These benefits are all IN ADDITION TO the benefits we are already receiving from intermittent fasting.

It is an often said—but an extremely accurate—truism that our lives are increasingly sedentary. One of the best ways to get exercise is to fit it into our everyday lives. Walk instead of drive; do some strength-building exercises when we get up in the morning.

If we drive to work, park the car at the end of the parking lot rather than by the entrance to your office. Stroll out to a shop to get lunch or fit in a walk during your lunch break. Exercise releases endorphins and fresh air awaken the brain – we find our afternoon performance is much improved if we have exercised during the middle of the day.

But exercise and intermittent fasting are not just two things we can do that is good for us. Most modern thinking agrees that there is a link between fasting and exercise which provides additional benefits for all the things we seek to achieve with the two activities.

The sum of combining the two is greater than the individual benefits they each offer. That is synergy. With fasting and exercise combined, 2 + 2 equals 5!

We burn more calories, see better internal cell repair, see greater mental health benefits. This is because modern thinking is challenging the age-old belief that we should not exercise on an empty stomach.

When our parents told us, as children, not to swim in the sea after eating lunch, they were speaking more sense than they intended; exercise-wise, a swim before lunch would have offered much better results (not that we probably needed to worry as children). What the latest research is showing us that it is better to exercise on an empty stomach.

To conclude this section: if we exercise during our fast, the total benefit is greater than the sum of its separate parts.

The best exercise to enhance the advantages of Fasting

To get a little (but not too) scientific for a moment, the speed at which we burn fat is determined by our sympathetic nervous system (SNS). Two things stimulate our SNS – one is the exercise itself, the other is not having a stomach full of food.

Thus, when we fast and exercise, we are initiating a combination of fat-burning pressures. But there are more –oxidative stress increases, which promotes muscle growth and strength. Leaner. Better. Stronger.

We can fine-tune this even more if we plan our exercise routines carefully.

Fasting Days: These should be used to undertake your low-intensity exercise. There are two reasons for this:

- if your sugar levels have fallen, then dizziness can strike with too much exercise,
- if the body is desperately looking for something to burn to create energy, it may attack muscle mass, which is something we want to keep.

Therefore, fasting days are great for doing walks, light swimming, and gentle jogs.

Non-Fasting Days: It is, therefore, logical that we save our high-intensity workouts for days when we have eaten. These are the times to hit the gym, to go for that long, hilly run, or to rip through our laps in the pool.

Weights: If weights form part of our exercise regime, then do this on our non-fasting days. Similarly, if we are looking for high-intensity short burst exercises, such as circuit training, non-fast days should be used. Also, with these types of workouts, we should eat, ideally within thirty minutes, after our exercise.

However, the joy of intermittent fasting for many people is that it is easy and flexible. For those on a serious weight loss or muscle building program, the advice above is necessary to achieve the results we seek. But for most of us, looking to get fitter, healthier, and a little lighter on our feet, it is enough to remember that any exercise is good for us, no matter what form it takes.

Chapter 7

Mistakes to avoid committing

Sticking to an intermittent fasting approach will let you experience tremendous benefits, among which are better digestion, significant weight loss, minimal sugar cravings, better sleep, and improved mental clarity. However, your journey towards attaining your desired results will most likely be accompanied by some errors. While you can't perfect intermittent fasting for the entire period you are planning to do it, take note that there are some mistakes committed by other practitioners of this eating pattern that you can simply avoid.

Mistake #1 – Changing your eating habits drastically

If you are one of those whose normal eating habits include eating every three to four hours or so then shrinking the time you need to eat within just 8 hours all of a sudden can lead to certain issues, like extreme hunger and frustration.

A lot of people make the mistake of adding drastic changes in their lifestyle and eating patterns all of a sudden by trying to stick to a long fasting period. This can lead to quitting after just a short period of fasting because they experienced difficulties in adjusting from their previous eating behaviors and habits.

You should avoid this mistake as much as possible if you want to succeed in IF.

Always remember that you might need around 10-14 days to finally adjust and prevent yourself from feeling extreme hunger during your fasting period. Avoid making the change in your eating habits all of a sudden. What you have to do, instead, is to stretch the amount of time in between your meals in a gradual manner (for instance, until you reach an eating window of 12 hours).

You should then move into an eating window of 10 hours. After that, reduce that window even further but only by small increments. Do this until you reached your target eating window.

Mistake #2 – Consuming the wrong liquids

Some people drink tea, black coffee, or water so they can go through their fasting period with the least amount of discomfort.

The problem is that if you can't tolerate black coffee then you may be tempted to add some sugar or milk without thinking about whether or not this will break your fast. Before adding anything to your drink, find out if it will affect your desired results first. If possible, do not let coconut oil and butter get near your coffee.

You should also stay away from liquids filled with protein, like bone broth. It is because these liquids can stop autophagy, which refers to a cellular process capable of breaking down and recycling damaged molecules. This is something that you may want to achieve when you are in your fasting period.

It is also advisable to stay away from diet sodas. You need to avoid anything, which is sweetened heavily, even those advertised as free of calories. Remember that even zero-calorie sweeteners can negatively affect your insulin level, which might also stimulate your appetite and cause cravings. To prevent taking in wrong liquids, keep track of your hydration and the specific drinks you take in.

This is a huge help in making yourself accountable and motivating yourself to stick to black coffee, plain tea, and water during the fasting period. Once you get used to drinking the right liquids, make sure that you do not forget to hydrate yourself, especially during the fasted state.

Note that while the IF regiment refrains you from eating foods during your fasting period, it is necessary for water or other healthy liquids to be close to you. It is mainly because this eating pattern might cause you to miss out on the kind of hydration often provided by healthy fruits and vegetables.

You do not want to suffer from dehydration as it has several side effects, like muscle cramps, hunger pangs, and headaches. With that in mind, ensure that you sip enough water and other allowed liquids throughout the day regardless if you are in your eating or fasting window.

Mistake #3 – Leading a sedentary lifestyle

Working out when you are sticking to the intermittent fasting approach might seem like a new endeavor for you, especially if you are used to eating a pre-workout snack. However, this should not be a reason why you should lead a sedentary lifestyle during your fasted state. Note that even if you are fasting, you can't still lose weight if you do not pair it with proper exercise.

The good news is that your body stores plenty of energy in your body fat. This is what your body will use in case there is no food. With that in mind, you can retain your usual exercise routines even when you have changed your eating pattern. If the entire experience is new then you may want to try out low-impact exercises, like walking.

In case you decide to fast overnight and work out during the morning then it is advisable to consume a meal rich in protein after it. It helps increase your body's muscle-building rate. One thing to remember before pairing IF with your regular workout, though, is that just like other exercise or diet plans, you have to consult your doctor first. However, in general, pairing your regular exercises with IF is safe.

Mistake #4 – Sticking to the wrong intermittent fasting plan or approach

Note that for IF to produce favorable results, you need to pick the right plan – one that perfectly fits your lifestyle, current condition, and personality. Avoid making yourself miserable by trying to stick to a pattern, which is not compatible with your lifestyle. If you know that you are a night owl, for instance, then avoid starting your fasting sessions every 6 pm.

In case you are someone who goes to the gym every day and does not want to sacrifice your daily workout then avoid picking an IF plan/method, which has severe calorie restrictions for several days every week. Consider your lifestyle and personality and find out which among the IF methods will work for you. By choosing the most suitable fasting method, it will be easier for you to stick to the new habit.

Mistake #5 – Beating yourself up in case you eat beyond your eating window

Do not feel too guilty if you slip up from the pattern sometimes. Avoid beating yourself up when you grab a food even if you are no longer in your eating window. Note that you need to listen to the cues sent by your body. If you feel real hunger then there is no reason to deprive yourself of what you need.

Remember that addressing your hunger is okay when doing intermittent fasting. Just make sure that you do not do it all the time. Also, one thing that you have to remind yourself constantly is that if you deny your body's hunger cues then your relationship with food will become unhealthy.

Do not be too hard on yourself and allow it to break from the fast in case you truly feel hungry during your supposed-to-be fasting state. Keep in mind that the idea behind intermittent fasting is not to starve yourself.

With that in mind, it is crucial to still provide yourself with the right nourishment, especially if you are starting to experience negative symptoms.

Mistake #6 – Restricting calories too much when the eating window comes

One problem experienced by those who just started following intermittent fasting is that the whole eating pattern causes them to continue restricting their calories even after breaking their fast.

You do not have to be too strict and rigid by excessively restricting your calorie intake. Note that intermittent fasting also requires you to hear what your body is telling you. Listen to it and eat until you experience fullness.

The good news is that the human body is actually an incredible machine but you also have to let it do its job correctly. In that case, you can expect it to release hormones that will let you know whether you are already full. You just have to watch out for the 1 it releases that signifies fullness.

Avoid restricting your calorie intake too much when you are supposed to eat. It is because doing so might only lead to under-eating, causing several unwanted body changes and long-term consequences.

Mistake #7 – Pushing yourself too hard

This is a mistake often committed by those who wish to try extending their fast for as long as possible even if it means forcing themselves. Some even go to the extent of fasting for more than 48 hours even if they already experience too much discomfort.

You should determine whether the extended/prolonged fast works for you before trying it out first.

Keep in mind that you can't expect the process of extending your fast to supercharge IF and produce more incredible benefits.

If you force yourself to fast for an extremely long period even to the point of extreme discomfort then consider seeking the help of a counselor whose specialty is on eating disorders.

The foods you regularly eat should not cause regret and remorse, so seeking the help of a professional can be beneficial.

Also, take note that your poor relationship with food can produce even bigger problems in the future. This is why talking to a counselor is advisable so you can figure out whether you already have an eating disorder or if your relationship with food is still healthy.

Mistake #8 – Obsessing over eating windows and schedules

One great benefit of intermittent fasting is that it teaches you to be fully in tune with your body signals. It allows you to understand real hunger, which is something that happens every 16 to 24 hours instead of every 4 hours that a lot of people believe.

With that in mind, you do not have to obsess too much over your eating windows and schedules.

You have to make sure that your body dictates the perfect time for you to eat, instead of the clock. Focusing on periods too much might cause you to count the hours left until your next meal. This will prevent you from learning and fully understanding the signals sent to you by your own body.

For instance, if you decide to skip breakfast then you are extending your fasting overnight to around 16 hours. Your focus should not be on the schedule or the time. This means that in case you decide to skip breakfast, then you also have the option of breaking the fast once you feel hungry, although it is advisable to do this only occasionally.

Mistake #9 – Trying to do numerous things at once

You may be forcing yourself to do a lot of things while trying to practice the intermittent fasting approach. Some of the things you might do are over-training, dry fasting, and under-eating.

Also, remember that if you are someone with poor eating habits and who lacks workout in the past and want to try intermittent fasting for better health then avoid biting more than what you can chew. This is important, especially if you are still a beginner.

Allow yourself to ease gradually into training and fasting. Also, avoid training 5 times weekly, fasting daily, and extremely restricting your calorie intake after fasting. It is because this might only trigger serious consequences in the future. One more thing to remind yourself is that your body survives with a bit of physical stress from time to time. However, you should try avoiding too much stress as this might produce more chronic issues.

Mistake #10 – Choosing the wrong foods

A lot of intermittent fasting followers also make the mistake of choosing the wrong foods. Many of those who tried it think that it is a magic pill capable of solving their weight and health problems.

While it is true that IF is an effective tool for those who want to have full control over their health and weight, it is still possible to cancel out its benefits if you eat the wrong foods, specifically processed and sugary ones, during your eating window.

Keep in mind that since you are fasting, it is more essential to give your body the right nourishment through whole and nutrient-dense foods. Being in the fasted state also encourages your body to break down any damaged parts then use these to produce energy. This is helpful in healing and cleansing your body.

This also results in the body becoming more and more sensitive to all the foods you take in. Such sensitivity is beneficial if you take in foods rich in nutrients.

However, it will not do you any good if the foods you consume do not nourish your body. If that is the case, you will experience extreme hunger most of the time since your body will start to crave nutrients. With that in mind, focus on consuming highly nutritious foods when it is already time to eat.

Do not just focus on cutting calories. Your goal is to ensure that your body still receives a sufficient amount of nutritious foods to ensure that your organs and your brain will continue to function well.

Intermittent Fasting myths

Intermittent fasting is one of the most rewarding eating patterns and lifestyles you can try. However, before starting your journey towards enjoying its numerous benefits, it is crucial to study the facts and myths behind it. This chapter will debunk some of the most famous intermittent fasting myths and offer truthful information about how this eating pattern works.

Myth #1 – Intermittent fasting guarantees significant weight loss

Contrary to what most people believe IF can't be expected to result in significant weight loss all the time. This is especially true if you are doing this approach the wrong way.

Note that regardless of the length of your fast, you can't still expect to achieve the results you want as far as weight loss is concerned if you constantly include burgers, candies, pizzas, and other unhealthy foods during your eating period. You still need to pair IF with regular exercise and a healthy diet. You can't treat each eating period as a cheat day.

Myth #2 – Intermittent fasting leads to muscle loss

No, your muscles will not shrivel up and break down during your fasted state. Keep in mind that the human body stores two forms of energy, namely fat and sugar. This means that your body will only be using these two forms of stored energy.

Protein, which is a major component of your muscles, will not be used by your body to produce energy when you are fasting. What happens, instead, is that your body will make use of sugar as the primary source of fuel during the first 1-2 days without food.

After that, your body will begin opening up and accessing stored fats as a source of energy. This means that it will start breaking down the stored fats in your body to create fuel once your stored sugar depletes. Each person has around 50,000 to 100,000 calories of fat on average stored in his body, which is equal to almost one month's worth of available stored fats.

If you intend to fast, therefore, then you do not have to worry about your muscles breaking down since it is your stored fat and sugar that your body will use as fuel.

Myth #3 – Intermittent fasting can slow down your metabolism

You do not have to worry about intermittent fasting negatively affecting your metabolic rate. It is because the entire eating pattern will not slow down your metabolism. Keep in mind that IF does not involve excessive calorie restrictions. What it does is to restrict the time you consume calories.

A few more hours spent waiting to take your first meal does not have a major effect on your metabolic rate. However, you should avoid under-eating during your eating period as this practice is the one that might send your metabolism downhill.

Myth #4 – Intermittent fasting can lead to poor brain performance

Glucose is your brain's main source of fuel. With that in mind, it is no longer surprising to see those who are planning to try IF worrying about being unable to give their brain a consistent supply of glucose. The truth, however, is that IF will not negatively affect the performance of your brain.

Keep in mind that your body is still capable of using stored fuel from your body to produce glucose. This means that even if you follow the low-carb intermittent fasting approach, it is still possible for your brain to get a good supply of fuel through ketone bodies that break down fat.

Intermittent fasting can even lead to better mental performance, focus, and clarity. It is mainly because fasting can stimulate epinephrine and norepinephrine production. If you get into the fasting mode, your body will cause a minor stress response, which releases adrenaline. This breaks down the fats stored in your body as fuel, thereby providing you with the focus and energy you need.

Furthermore, fasting can lead to the production of BDNF (brain-derived neurotrophic factor). This can help your existing neurons survive, stimulate the growth of new neurons, and improve your learning and thinking ability and memory. It also helps lessen your risk of suffering from depression and Alzheimer's disease.

Myth #5 – You have limitless options during your eating window

Some of those who tried intermittent fasting wrongly believed that they are allowed to eat whatever they want to be provided they consume it during the eating window.

This is not true. Eating without limitations during the eating window can only have serious consequences to your health, wellness, and weight loss goals. Eating anything during the eating period might cause your body to get confused.

It is because from being on a fasting state that results in balanced levels of blood glucose and fat burning, your body suddenly experiences a spike in insulin and blood glucose. If this happens, you are just basically ruining the incredible effort you have exerted for fasting.

Furthermore, not controlling the amount of food you eat during your eating window can make you feel terrible and produce issues, like weight gain, mood swings, and hormonal imbalance.

Note that while intermittent fasting does not require you to be extremely strict during your eating window, you still have to balance the foods you eat. It is still crucial to apply moderation as this can help you gather the results you want from IF.

Myth #6 – Intermittent fasting is the sole reason for macronutrient deficiency

Remember that if you follow your preferred intermittent fasting method the right way, you do not have to worry about experiencing a nutrient deficiency.

Fasting is not the main reason for nutrient deficiency. Diet plans that are deficient in nutrients are the culprit. You will not suffer from a nutrient deficiency if you stick to eating whole, balanced, and nutritious foods during your eating window.

You do not have to worry too much about your body not getting enough nutrients when you are fasting as there is no basis for such a claim. Fasting can cause your body to create nutrient efficiency. It increases the possibility of your body utilizing fewer nutrients, thereby retaining them so your body can efficiently use them in the future.

With that in mind, fasting can't be pointed to as the culprit for nutrient deficiency but poor diet, chronic stress, unstable blood sugar levels, leaky gut syndrome, and low levels of stomach acid.

Myth #7 – Intermittent fasting can lead to overeating

This is not true. What dictates your unhealthy eating behavior includes leptin and blood sugar. Having unstable blood sugar levels can cause food cravings, especially if your sugar crashes down. Being desensitized to leptin can also result in difficulties in figuring out whether you have already consumed enough foods.

Leptin refers to a signaling hormone within your body, which plays a huge role in controlling your hunger. Certain factors, like chronic calorie restriction, poor quality of sleep, binge eating, and stress can lead to leptin resistance, causing you to be at a higher risk of overeating.

Instead of causing you to overeat, intermittent fasting can stabilize your blood sugar and improve your sensitivity to leptin. This can further improve your ability to control overeating or binge eating.

Myth #8 – You won't be able to exercise if you are fasting

This is a misconception since it is safe for you to exercise even if you are in your fasting period. Working out will not result in muscle wasting or loss. Fast workouts can lead to the growth of your muscles provided you still consume adequate amounts of protein and calories every day.

Besides, working out while fasting can also produce other incredible benefits, including improved ketosis state, better fat-burning ability, and increased growth hormone levels.

Just make sure to stay hydrated if you intend to do some high-intensity exercises during your fasting state. In case you wish to gain muscles, then it would be helpful to take essential amino acid supplements.

Myth #9 – Intermittent fasting can lead to starving and irritability

A lot of those who haven't tried intermittent fasting yet but want to do it for health reasons are often concerned about getting irritable if they experience extreme hunger. While this statement bears some weight, note that it is only true temporarily.

You may experience irritability and hunger at first, especially if you are used to eating at least three meals spaced periodically every day. This may happen because you are still adjusting to your new eating routine/pattern.

You can't expect this to happen permanently, though. You can slowly make the adjustments by doing simple fasting routines or by doing it one to two times every week at first. This will allow you to introduce the routine to your system. You can then slowly increase the number and duration of your fasting sessions as soon as you feel comfortable.

You do not have to rush things. Allow your body to adapt so you will not end up experiencing too much hunger and irritability. Once you are fully adjusted to this eating pattern, you can start enjoying its numerous benefits like better mental clarity and mood.

Myth #10 – Intermittent fasting does not work for those suffering from diabetes

Another myth associated with fasting that you have to be aware of is that it is ineffective for diabetics. It is because most people are made to believe that they need to consume foods constantly as a means of maintaining their blood sugar level.

The truth, however, is that IF works for those suffering from Type 2 diabetes, especially in improving weight loss results and stabilizing blood sugar.

Prolonged fasting even can restore their insulin sensitivity. You may also combine IF with a ketogenic diet if you want to further improve its ability to restore your sensitivity to insulin. What is good about having improved insulin sensitivity is that your body will no longer need to produce too much insulin. This results in minimal inflammation, which is a big help for diabetics and those who are prone to developing kidney and heart diseases.

Type 1 diabetes sufferers who are incapable of producing insulin, however, should closely keep track of their blood sugar level before practicing intermittent fasting so they can do it correctly. They can still fast for around 12-16 hours every day but this will depend on the stability of their blood sugar level.

Chapter 8

Side effects of Intermittent Fasting

While intermittent fasting is one of the most beneficial eating patterns that you can try at present, you still need to be extremely cautious before starting. Keep in mind that it is not risk-free. This makes it necessary to talk to your physician first and find out whether it is safe for you to follow this style of eating.

Also, find out if you have any health problems or complications that might cause the negative side effects, instead of rewarding benefits, of intermittent fasting to come out. It also helps to understand the most common side effects of intermittent fasting so you can study the whole approach carefully and find out how you can avoid them as much as possible.

- Tiredness – When doing IF, there is a high risk for you to experience tiredness and grogginess, especially if you are still a beginner. Take note that in this situation, your body will also most likely run on less energy than what it is used to. Fasting might also increase your stress level and disrupt your normal sleep patterns. To avoid this specific side effect of intermittent fasting, it would be helpful for you to meditate or do other activities that will lower your stress levels. If you are working out regularly, then consider scheduling it during your eating period. This helps conserve your energy. Besides, keep in mind that exercising while you are in a fast state might lower your blood sugar level, which can trigger symptoms, like confusion and dizziness. It helps to be on the safe side by working out when you have already eaten.
- Headaches – You may be dealing with headaches because your body will tend to adjust to your new eating pattern. It could be caused by dehydration so it is advisable to drink plenty of water both during your eating window and fasting period. You may also experience headaches due to a

sudden drop in your blood sugar level and the release of stress hormones during the fasting period. The good news is that headaches usually happen only because your body is still in the adjustment stage. This means that this side effect is not permanent. Once you get used to it, you will no longer suffer from headaches.

- Heartburn – You may also experience heartburn due to fasting. In most cases, this problem will be resolved after around a couple of months. It is necessary to visit and consult your doctor in case your heartburn does not seem to resolve on its own even after your body has adjusted to the new eating pattern. Heartburn is often a result of your unfamiliarity with the fasting scenario, causing your body to release stomach acids automatically at certain times. While this can cause discomfort, this only happens at the beginning of your journey so there is no need for you to worry too much about it.
- Brain fog – This is also another common side effect of intermittent fasting, especially if your body is not yet used to the habit of not eating. This might cause your mind to try keeping up with the new routine, leading to confusion, forgetfulness, or brain fog. Once you familiarize yourself with how IF works, though, and your body has adjusted to the habit, you can expect better brain function from fasting.
- Diarrhea – Another unpleasant side effect of IF is diarrhea and it usually happens to those who are still beginners in fasting. There is an even higher risk for you to experience this problem if you enter the fasting period after consuming too many carbs. This problem may be associated with a significant drop in your insulin level, signaling your kidneys to get rid of excess water. This is the reason why you might experience unwanted and watery bowel movements. You

should also remember that your body tends to lose electrolytes via bowel movements and urination. If you experience watery stools or diarrhea, then one sign that you may experience at first is a low level of sodium. With that in mind, it helps to drink broth or pickle juice during those days when you are dealing with this uncomfortable and unwanted IF side effect. It also helps to add around 1-2 pinches of salt in the water you drink.

- Insomnia and anxiety – Both these side effects may be caused by the production of adrenaline, a counter-regulatory hormone when you begin to fast. In most cases, this effect is beneficial as it results in a high metabolic rate and energy level. The problem is that the energy you get from it might be too high even during those specific times when you are supposed to be sleeping. This can also make you feel jittery and anxious. It could be because of consuming too much coffee especially during the beginning of your fasting journey. Your anxiety also tends to worsen if you constantly worry about the effects of fasting on your health. You can resolve these side effects by sticking to proper bedtime routines, such as turning off your gadgets and electronics ninety minutes before your bedtime. You can also relax with the help of Epsom salt baths.
- Bad breath – Another unpleasant and unexpected side effect of intermittent fasting is bad breath. This often happens if you already start losing weight due to fasting. This side effect is also referred to as the keto breath characterized by your tongue becoming white and a taste of acetone in your mouth. It is mainly because acetone is known as the by-product of metabolizing fatty acid. A lot of those who tried fasting and experienced the keto breath tend to freak out upon noticing their white tongues. They even wrongly assume that it is a result of nutrient

deficiency. If this happens to you then avoid freaking out. This is your body's normal reaction to the fat-burning process. As weight loss starts slowing down, you will notice a great improvement in your breath. You will also notice your tongue going back to its normal pink color. If you feel uncomfortable with this side effect then there are some things that you can do to manage it. One is to brush your teeth as frequently as possible throughout the day. Drinking more water and using a tongue scraper can also help. Intermittent fasting provides numerous benefits to those who are obese, overweight, and have average weight. However, it is not appropriate for everyone, including pregnant and breastfeeding women and those who are dealing with eating disorders and certain health issues.

This is the main reason why you have to study the effects of fasting on you as soon as you begin doing it. Listen to your own body. If you notice some unwanted side effects, find out if it is because your body is just adjusting to the routine or due to more serious issues. If you are extremely worried about the negative side effects, do not hesitate to consult your doctor to ensure your safety.

Sample routine

A 16/8 sample routine can be designed in a trillion number of ways with a variety of options of what to eat when to eat, and how to eat. The individuals we will be designing the sample routine for are working people with regular jobs with free time on the weekends.

What is the routine of an average job person? He or she wakes up, takes a shower, cooks and has breakfast, leaves for the office by 8 am depending on whether the person has a car or has to walk, works till 5 to 6 pm, and reaches home at night for dinner. Fasting during such a tight and hectic schedule will not be an easy decision to make until everything is planned according to your comfort zone.

Let's set up a 7-day intermittent fasting routine for a beginner who has a job to handle and can only party on weekends. We shall start with 12 hours fast and increase it to 16 hours by the end of the week. Skipping meals is completely optional, but we will adjust it according to the routine of our workaholic individual.

Number of Days	Day 1	Day 2	Day 3	Day 4	Day 5	Day 6	Day 7
Fasting window (in hours)	12	13	14	15	16	16	16
Feeding window (in hours)	12	11	10	9	8	8	8

Such a table can be really helpful to adapt to the 16/ 8 fasting method quickly with just a 1-hour increase in the fasting window.

Here's a brief idea of what one's eating window should look like, and the kind of foods portions that suit a 16:8 fasting diet.

Morning eating window:

- 8 am: an egg, scrambled, boiled, baked, or an omelet with green veggies, corn, olives, and mushrooms;
- Midnight: avocadoes, apples, berries, bananas, or any other citrus fruits that you like and are available;
- 3 to 4 pm: veggie stir-fried or boiled vegetables with chicken breast;
- during the evening: black coffee or decaf tea.

Afternoon eating window:

- morning green tea, warm water, black coffee or tea;
- 11 am peanut butter banana smoothie;
- 2 pm: nuts garnished on avocado toast;

- 4 pm: cashew nuts, almonds, and pistachios;
- 7 pm: rich tomato sauce over whole wheat ravioli or pasta with meatballs.

Late eating or evening window:

- morning green tea, warm water, black coffee or tea;
- 1 pm: berry chia seed pudding with a granola bar and yogurt;
- 4 pm: carrots and hummus;
- 9 pm: grilled fish or salmon, veggies, and quinoa.

You are not restricted to have these very meals; these are just examples of how light your meals and snacks should be and how you can divide the eating window into small meal portions with intervals.

However, all the food items mentioned in this diet plan include nutrient-dense food and are mentioned in sufficient quantities to provide you with energy for the entire day. This is just an example of keeping in mind the eating windows. Later the importance of warm water will also be signified.

The intake of water and fluids also have suitable times, and when we tell you these minute details make a difference, know that it will take the spotlight. If you skip breakfast, you will be following the mid-day eating window.

If you skip dinner you will practice the late-evening eating window, and if you are planning to skip lunch you will have to follow both the early morning and late evening window. However, what I feel goes best with the workers' point of view will depend on the kind of work they are doing, physical exertion or mental exertion, or both.

For a person who has a job, he or requires energy during the day. Therefore, they should fast at night so that most of the fasting period is spent sleeping. Keep the fast as fun as you can, kill boredom, do it your way and complete the challenge. Let's kill it!

Monday to Friday being weekdays will follow a routine of the typical working days.

Day 1 (Monday) On Monday, we start with a 12-hour fasting window with a 12 hour feeding time frame. This is the smallest time frame kept in the entire week. Get started and understand the intermittent fasting schedule so that you can adapt to the changes in the upcoming days. Prepare your body and brain for the new eating style and habits.

Start the day by skipping breakfast every day starting from day 1 to day 5. This is not at all unhealthy and is just a myth that was started by breakfast related item companies to promote their sales. Also, you are not skipping a meal technically; instead, you are just pushing its eating time a little forward.

This way you do not trigger your insulin levels early morning. Prefer having a glass of warm mineral water with or without a splash of lemon on an empty stomach as you wake up. It does amazing wonders, and this research is published in the European Journal of Pharmaceutical and Medical Research.

Physicians recommend that such a strategy lessens any free radical activity going on within the body, cleanses the digestion process, helps in constipation, acts as the super-natural home remedy for pain and cramps, improves blood circulation, and sheds excess pounds. You can say that it is a weight loss technique in its self.

On the other hand, cold water slows down your metabolism and does not consist of vital minerals. Keep your water intake high as it will burn your appetite and reduce any temptations.

After the water intake, you can go for a cup of black coffee or tea if you desire. You can consume no-calorie drinks until your fast ends.

Break the fast exactly at midnight and have your first meal of the day with satiating foods or nutrient-dense foods. It's important to feed yourself properly during your eating window. If the afternoon eating window matches your taste buds, go for it or else you can take reference from the following:

- meal 1 at midnight: chia pudding with any fruit of your choice;
- meal 2 at 5 pm: Chinese chicken salad or Caesar salad with your favorite toppings and protein bar as a snack;
- meal 3 at 10 pm: spicy chicken curry with brown rice.

For the 12-hour eating window, there is a huge gap between every meal which is good as the food you have eaten gets digested, but it is not considered a crime if you are craving some snacks.

You can eat as much as you desire during this window, but it's better to stay on the 3 nutrient-rich meals. Note down the number of calories you have consumed for day 1.

You might be in your office during the first two meal consumption times, so exercising may not be possible. To keep your metabolism active, you need to stay active. Although you have to maintain discipline, know that the struggle has just begun.

It's good if you can spend an hour at the gym on your way back home. The workout will tighten your muscles and prepare your body for the final meal. It will also keep you fresh and boost your metabolism.

Keep the workout routine normal and not intense as it is your first day. Build your stamina and then move to power training. You do not want to eat the same menu every day, and that is completely fine, so you can make the alterations as you like.

Just make sure to have nutrient-dense foods.

If you have protein in the form of a protein bar one day, have it in the form of beef on the next day, a protein shake, or an egg later. Fruits are the best source of vitamin c, and vegetables of iron, fiber, and vitamins.

The chia seeds act as a fulfilling and yummy dessert, yet healthy and low in carbohydrates. After breaking your fast at 8 pm, watch television or Netflix for a while, enter into a relaxing mode and sleep early. These diet routines require a minimum of 7-hour sleep.

This will promote a healthy lifestyle, stop you from binge eating, or having late-night cravings while improving metabolism with better weight maintenance and reduction in the risk of heart diseases.

It also prevents your brain from staying confused the entire night on whether to keep telling you to sleep or to stay awake as a tired body resists sleep.

Day 2 (Tuesday) We now have increased our fasting window by an hour, making it 13 hours for fasting and 11 hours of feeding.

These 11 hours will start the same as day 1 with the same routine, but a different meal. To keep it short, wake up, have warm water, and fast with low-calorie drinks till midnight, break your fast at midnight and start feeding yourself:

- meal 1 at midnight: mint protein shakes with nuts for snacking;
- meal 2 at 5 pm: feta cheese salad and fruits of your choice (best suggestions remain citrus fruits, apples, bananas, and berries);

meal 3 at 9 pm: beans with brown rice or bread or lentils and hummus. Snacking is allowed in between the eating window, but it is your second day today, therefore start taking things seriously.

Cut on your carbohydrates and switch to a high protein diet. Understand what intermittent fasting is all about and remember the tested theories so that you can practice it deeply. Get your jogger laces tight as you need to tighten your workout routines.

Keep your caffeine fluids on the go to feel less hungry during the day. Also, the "right time" to drink water to contribute to weight loss is the moment you wake up, before the meal, before taking a bath, and before going to bed.

It's good to keep yourself hydrated all the time. You should drink water at least half an hour before having your meal to let your body suck the nutrients.

You can also have water after the meal, but a minimum of an hour later to let your food digest properly. Do not drink ice-cold water though, even if it's extremely hot.

Day 3 (Wednesday) With the onset of the third day, the fast increases to 14 hours with a 10-hour eating window:

- meal 1 at midnight: poached eggs with spinach and almonds and yogurt for snacking;
- meal 2 at 4 pm: tuna salad sandwiches;
- meal 3 at 9 pm: Asian fried rice.

Now stop and appreciate yourself by rewarding yourself for reaching this point. The reward may be putting a cross on the number of days that have gone or an expensive one, like a dinner.

You can collect tokens for this reward. With every successful intermittent fast, you reward yourself one token, and as soon as the token reaches 5, you can go out for dinner.

These rewards will make your connection with this routine stronger and inform your brain that you are enjoying and not facing any hurdles in your way.

Day 4 (Thursday) Finally, you are reaching your target time eating window. For Thursday you have a 15 hour fast and a 9-hour eating window. Have you started changing your eating habits? Follow:

- meal 1 at midnight: egg muffins and fruits of your choice;
- meal 2 at 4 pm: broccoli salad with dark chocolate and nuts for nibbling;
- meal 3 at 9 pm: lemon-flavored garlic grilled beef and green tea.

This day was your high protein day. It was necessary to slowly bring you to a high protein diet so that you can get used to it sooner. You might feel heavy after dinner, so it will be best if you have a cup of green tea and go for a slow walk. Wait for 2 to 3 hours to let your food digest and then sleep.

Day 5 (Friday) Now your fast has finally reached the 16/8 protocol, and you are officially ready to rock the routine. To be honest, the day will be difficult to handle at the start but keep a winning mindset. You can do this!

Increase your intake of black coffee from now onwards as it has antioxidants that double your metabolism and suppress your diet too.

Reminder: Your eating window is only 6 hours now, so do not forget or skip a meal because starving will not be accepted and will not aid in weight loss. Remember to have more protein, more water, black coffee, and exercise. Use this pattern:

- meal 1 at midnight: bagel and cream cheese sandwich, nuts or snack;
- meal 2 at 3 pm: Caesar salad with olive oil dressing, fruit for a snack;
- meal 3 at 6 pm: lentils with beans can be very healthy and a glass of warm milk.

Warm milk before sleep will help you sleep better, and a minimum of seven-hour sleep is vital to support this diet routine. An empty stomach can trouble you at night. This is scientifically proven and also has been mentioned in the research of a student from the

University of Waterloo, that milk contains tryptophan, which is a sleep inducer naturally.

A study published in the British Medical Journal took 18 people under observation with 10 young and 8 old adults.

They were given Horlicks before sleeping, and the results concluded that the 8 adults had a good sound sleep with no periods of wakefulness.

The other 10 were a little restless though. You must be thinking of when to drink the milk if the fast ends at 6 pm.

You can also shift the window from 12 pm to 6 pm or 3 pm to 9 pm. This way you can enjoy an outing with a fine dining dinner too, but do not make this a ritual and cheat on your diet.

Day 6 (Saturday) It is the weekend guys! It's time to chill out a little, but with the weekend vibe, not following the diet routine. We all have plans with family and friends as the weekend approaches.

With these get-togethers, come lots of drama, gossip and obviously "the food". We are always up for a party, but what about intermitting fasting? You must be sad, but not to worry as remember the 90/10 cheat rule. It's fine to have a little high-calorie food for a meal within your eating window if you keep the calorie count.

This is your schedule:

- meal 1 at 3 pm: boiled eggs with orange juice;
- meal 2 at 6 pm: cabbage, tomato or garlic corn soup or Thai citrus salad with dark chocolate for a snack;
- meal 3 at 9 pm: anything at the gathering or party.

You can interchange meal 1 and meal 2 according to the time and day of the event you will be visiting. On the weekend, you will have enough free time to focus on your exercises. Go for a morning jog and do an intense workout at the gym.

Day 7 (Sunday) Finally, we have successfully reached the end of the week. Let's ace these 16 hours today, and then continue the routine till it becomes a habit. Here we go:

- meal 1 at 2 pm: coconut protein balls;
- meal 2 at 5 pm: Taco salad;
- meal 3 at 8 pm: whole wheat chapatti with cooked vegetables in olive oil or roasted beef with seasoning.

One last and very typical, yet important thing to mention is, "Do not let boredom stress you out." Getting bored can be your enemy at this stage as it leads to stress, which will make you depressed and lead to anxiety. This will also create a hormonal imbalance and make you a lazy person planning to give up sooner or later.

This way intermittent fasting would not help you lose weight. Therefore, you need to stay busy. We are done for the week, and I have to say that you did great. Keep up the good work and make yourself proud.

Workout at the gym as if you own it, and eat smartly. Ace that weight loss target, and maintain it with confidence.

30 Days Meal-Plan to help you while on IF 16/8

The 16:8 intermittent fasting method is the most popular choice because it tends to be the easiest one to follow.

Since it is the most popular, and it will more than likely be the one that you choose to follow, I am going to provide you with a 30-day schedule for the 16:8 protocol.

It's not so much a challenge as it is a schedule to help you get started with your intermittent fasting diet. I will put times in this schedule, but you can easily change them to suit your personal needs. The point is that you will reduce your eating window to eight hours.

You are also allowed to eat whatever foods and beverages you like during that eight-hour window, and as many meals, as you want.

The schedule below will provide you with a sample menu to help you out with some healthier options, though.

You don't have to restrict your calorie intake either, but it is recommended that you:

- Eat a certain combination of different foods that provide you with lots of nutrients, such as vegetables and fruits, high-fiber whole grains, lean protein, and healthy fats.
- Consume at least the recommended amount of water during the day. This includes the hours where you don't get to eat as well. Water is a freebie in every diet.

This challenge will also give you an eight-minute exercise routine that you can do before your first meal of the day to help boost the effects of the fast. This workout is comprised of cardio and resistance training intervals. Without further ado, here is your 30-Day 16:8 intermittent fasting protocol.

Day 1

- Wake Up – Coffee, green tea, or zero-calorie detox drink.
- Breakfast 1 PM – Scrambled eggs with toast.
- Snack 2:30 PM – 1 serving of almonds and an orange.
- Dinner 8 PM – Grilled chicken and veggies and bread pudding for dessert.

Day 2

- Wake Up – Coffee, green tea, or zero-calorie detox drink.
- Breakfast 1 PM – Avocado toast with tomato, bacon, and egg.
- Snack 2:30 PM – cucumber and watermelon salad.
- Dinner 8 PM – Baked fish and veggies and ice cream for dessert.

Day 3

- Wake Up – Coffee, green tea, or zero-calorie detox drink.
- Breakfast 1 PM – Kale, banana, and peanut butter smoothie.
- Snack 2:30 PM – Medium-sized dark chocolate brownie.
- Dinner 8 PM – Asian style chicken soup and fruit custard for dessert.

Day 4

- Wake Up – Coffee, green tea, or zero-calorie detox drink.
- Breakfast 1 PM – Breakfast sandwich on whole-wheat toast.
- Snack 2:30 PM – Serving of mixed nuts.
- Dinner 8 PM – Kidney bean chili with two to three chapattis, and a dark chocolate brownie for dessert.

Day 5

- Wake Up – Coffee, green tea, or zero-calorie detox drink.
- Breakfast 1 PM – Tofu scramble with tomato.
- Snack 2:30 PM – 4 almonds and an apple.
- Dinner 8 PM – Grilled chicken and veggies and ice cream for dessert.

Day 6

- Wake Up – Coffee, green tea, or zero-calorie detox drink.
- Breakfast 1 PM – Scrambled eggs with peanut butter toast.
- Snack 2:30 PM – Small bowl of nachos with a low-fat dip.
- Dinner 8 PM – Vegetable lasagna with bread pudding for dessert.

Day 7

- Wake Up – Coffee, green tea, or zero-calorie detox drink.
- Breakfast 1 PM – Bacon and eggs with whole wheat toast.

- Snack 2:30 PM – 1 serving of almonds and an orange.
- Dinner 8 PM – Tuna sandwich with a low-fat milkshake for dessert.

Day 8

- Wake Up – Coffee, green tea, or zero-calorie detox drink.
- Breakfast 1 PM – Wheat flakes and milk.
- Snack 2:30 PM – 1 serving of mixed nuts.
- Dinner 8 PM – Grilled chicken tortilla wrap and bread pudding for dessert.

Day 9

- Wake Up – Coffee, green tea, or zero-calorie detox drink.
- Breakfast 1 PM – Kale, strawberry, and blueberry smoothie.
- Snack 2:30 PM – Cucumber and watermelon salad.
- Dinner 8 PM – Kidney bean chili and fruit custard for dessert.

Day 10

- Wake Up – Coffee, green tea, or zero-calorie detox drink.
- Breakfast 1 PM – Scrambled eggs with toast.
- Snack 2:30 PM – A medium-sized dark chocolate brownie
- Dinner 8 PM – Baked fish and veggies with low-fat frozen yogurt for dessert.

Day 11

- Wake Up – Coffee, green tea, or zero-calorie detox drink.
- Breakfast 1 PM – Avocado toast with sliced chicken breast and tomato.
- Snack 2:30 PM – Apple and watermelon.
- Dinner 8 PM – Grilled chicken and veggie kebab with ice cream for dessert.

Day 12

- Wake Up – Coffee, green tea, or zero-calorie detox drink.
- Breakfast 1 PM – Breakfast sandwich on whole-wheat toast.
- Snack 2:30 PM – A small bowl of nachos with a low-fat dip.
- Dinner 8 PM – Buffalo chicken tortilla wrap with a fresh fruit salad for dessert.

Day 13

- Wake Up – Coffee, green tea, or zero-calorie detox drink.
- Breakfast 1 PM – Scrambled eggs with peanut butter toast.
- Snack 2:30 PM – A small bowl of potato wafers.
- Dinner 8 PM – Indian lentil soup with fruit custard for dessert.

Day 14

- Wake Up – Coffee, green tea, or zero-calorie detox drink.
- Breakfast 1 PM – Curried tofu scramble.
- Snack 2:30 PM – 4 almonds and an apple.
- Dinner 8 PM – Baked chicken with roasted vegetables and a side salad with a dark chocolate brownie for dessert.

Day 15

- Wake Up – Coffee, green tea, or zero-calorie detox drink.
- Breakfast 1 PM – Bacon, egg, avocado, and whole-wheat toast.
- Snack 2:30 PM – Cucumber and watermelon salad.
- Dinner 8 PM – Vegetable lasagna with a low-fat milkshake for dessert.

Day 16

- Wake Up – Coffee, green tea, or zero-calorie detox drink.
- Breakfast 1 PM – Scrambled eggs with toast.
- Snack 2:30 PM – 4 almonds and an orange.

- Dinner 8 PM – Grilled chicken and veggies and bread pudding for dessert.

Day 17

- Wake Up – Coffee, green tea, or zero-calorie detox drink.
- Breakfast 1 PM – Avocado toast with tomato, bacon, and egg.
- Snack 2:30 PM – cucumber and watermelon salad.
- Dinner 8 PM – Baked fish and veggies and ice cream for dessert.

Day 18

- Wake Up – Coffee, green tea, or zero-calorie detox drink.
- Breakfast 1 PM – Kale, banana, and peanut butter smoothie.
- Snack 2:30 PM – Medium-sized dark chocolate brownie.
- Dinner 8 PM – Asian style chicken soup and fruit custard for dessert.

Day 19

- Wake Up – Coffee, green tea, or zero-calorie detox drink.
- Breakfast 1 PM – Breakfast sandwich on whole-wheat toast.
- Snack 2:30 PM – Small bowl of popcorn.
- Dinner 8 PM – Kidney bean chili with two to three chapattis, and a dark chocolate brownie for dessert.

Day 20

- Wake Up – Coffee, green tea, or zero-calorie detox drink.
- Breakfast 1 PM – Tofu scramble with tomato.
- Snack 2:30 PM – 4 almonds and an apple.
- Dinner 8 PM – Grilled chicken and veggies and ice cream for dessert.

Day 21

- Wake Up – Coffee, green tea, or zero-calorie detox drink.
- Breakfast 1 PM – Scrambled eggs with peanut butter toast.
- Snack 2:30 PM – Small bowl of nachos with a low-fat dip.
- Dinner 8 PM – Vegetable lasagna with bread pudding for dessert.

Day 22

- Wake Up – Coffee, green tea, or zero-calorie detox drink.
- Breakfast 1 PM – Bacon and eggs with whole wheat toast.
- Snack 2:30 PM – 4 almonds and an orange.
- Dinner 8 PM – Tuna sandwich with a low-fat milkshake for dessert.

Day 23

- Wake Up – Coffee, green tea, or zero-calorie detox drink.
- Breakfast 1 PM – Wheat flakes and milk.
- Snack 2:30 PM – Small bowl of popcorn.
- Dinner 8 PM – Grilled chicken tortilla wrap and bread pudding for dessert.

Day 24

- Wake Up – Coffee, green tea, or zero-calorie detox drink.
- Breakfast 1 PM – Kale, strawberry, and blueberry smoothie.
- Snack 2:30 PM – Cucumber and watermelon salad.
- Dinner 8 PM – Kidney bean chili and fruit custard for dessert.

Day 25

- Wake Up – Coffee, green tea, or zero-calorie detox drink.
- Breakfast 1 PM – Scrambled eggs with toast.
- Snack 2:30 PM – A medium-sized dark chocolate brownie

- Dinner 8 PM – Baked fish and veggies with low-fat frozen yogurt for dessert.

Day 26

- Wake Up – Coffee, green tea, or zero-calorie detox drink.
- Breakfast 1 PM – Avocado toast with sliced chicken breast and tomato.
- Snack 2:30 PM – Apple and watermelon.
- Dinner 8 PM – Grilled chicken and veggie kebab with ice cream for dessert.

Day 27

- Wake Up – Coffee, green tea, or zero-calorie detox drink.
- Breakfast 1 PM – Breakfast sandwich on whole-wheat toast.
- Snack 2:30 PM – A small bowl of nachos with a low-fat dip.
- Dinner 8 PM – Buffalo chicken tortilla wrap with a fresh fruit salad for dessert.

Day 28

- Wake Up – Coffee, green tea, or zero-calorie detox drink.
- Breakfast 1 PM – Scrambled eggs with peanut butter toast.
- Snack 2:30 PM – A small bowl of potato wafers.
- Dinner 8 PM – Indian lentil soup with fruit custard for dessert.

Day 29

- Wake Up – Coffee, green tea, or zero-calorie detox drink.
- Breakfast 1 PM – Curried tofu scramble.
- Snack 2:30 PM – 4 almonds and an apple.
- Dinner 8 PM – Baked chicken with roasted vegetables and a side salad with a dark chocolate brownie for dessert.

Day 30

- Wake Up – Coffee, green tea, or zero-calorie detox drink.
- Breakfast 1 PM – Bacon, egg, avocado, and whole-wheat toast.
- Snack 2:30 PM – Cucumber and watermelon salad.
- Dinner 8 PM – Vegetable lasagna with a low-fat milkshake for dessert.

Hacks to help you succeed

There are many principal tips and tricks that I use to this day to continue to ensure my success. While intermittent fasting is all about the timing of your meals and fasting, it can be so much more if you decide to use it. Intermittent fasting along with the hacks discussed below will change your weight and your life forever.

Remaining motivated on the path of weight loss can be tough or challenging at times. Losing weight is a lonely road.

People may praise you for the improvements you make, but no one is there to share your trials and tribulations. The pains and gains of the weight loss journey always stay with you.

Weight loss journeys can be disappointing and painful at times. There may come times when you would want to put your guard down. There are points of disillusionment in the life of almost everyone passing through this journey where he/she starts feeling the whole process futile and worthless.

It is not the journey that becomes worthless; it is our mind trying to find an excuse to get out of the tough situation. It is simply a reaction of fight or flight response.

You must stay strong and motivated. These times are painful, but they pass away very quickly. You must draw inspiration from people around you, and take support from the people near and dear to you.

The best way to survive and thrive on this path is to find your support pillars. You can draw support from the following:

Friends and Family. This is the natural support base for everyone. It is a reliable support base you can look up to. You must confide in them as it gives you power. You can share your victories and failures with them, and hence, nothing keeps building inside you. You will always find yourself as light as a feather.

Sharing your problems or challenges with family and friends also helps in avoiding uncomfortable situations. If you are trying to avoid eating a certain type of food, the family members can avoid bringing or eating it in front of you. The atmosphere remains more empathetic.

Support Groups. You find people suffering from the same problems in support groups, and hence, you can relate to them and share your problems with them easily. Support groups play a great role in removing inhibitions.

People don't feel strange, and they are better able to answer each other's questions. Most people have been through similar situations; hence, it is easier to find people with common struggles.

Professionals. You can also take the help of professionals like doctors, dieticians, nutritionists. They are better equipped to answer your technical queries, and they can guide you in the right direction. If you are already suffering from any chronic illness, then you must seek the help of a professional; as regular monitoring of the problem is important for your very own safety.

Sharing is Caring. I am not certain if this will help anyone other than myself or not, but it did help and is still helping me. I have learned that I am best at all things in life when I am helping others along the way. I have been sharing my knowledge with people day in and day and have become a coach of intermittent fasting to many.

By encouraging others, I have simultaneously helped myself, because it's a shame to teach what you can't follow right? I won't be that type of coach. I practice what I am teaching. Me writing this book has helped me learn that I know so much about this topic, which is why I have been so much more successful this time around.

I gain so much pleasure from my social media follower's interest in my story and growth. I have so much respect from my coworkers and friends and they all ask so many questions about IF, so literally this is all I talk about, which is fine by me, it holds me accountable.

I don't want to let myself down to include a lot of people who are seamlessly watching me out of the corner of their eyes. I am helping someone else with this knowledge, which helps me.

Apps to Download. Pinterest is such a good resource to use when it comes to planning meals to keep eating the healthier way.

This app includes links to recipes, grocery lists, meal ideas, how to prep these meals, and more. YouTube, of course, is a great resource to review other people's struggles, peaks, and pits, before and after pictures, to hear their stories, to help you stay motivated and understand that most of what you go through while attempting to make this a habit, others have gone through the same things.

MyFitnessPal's blog and community sections of its app is another great resource to use to join communities that are specific to intermittent fasting and all its components.

These are good apps to have downloaded on your mobile device, iPad, or tablet. Using all your free time on these apps should be your new hobby instead of scrolling on your social media, especially since everything you see and hear will contribute to the success of making intermittent fasting a hobby.

Food Delivery Services. Some people decide that Meal Planning and Meal Prep is just not a realistic lifestyle for them. They may live a busier life than average, have a big active family, hate to cook, can't cook, don't want to cook, hate shopping, not creative, and more reasons.

These people may choose to use a meal planning/prep or food delivery service to assist them with their meals. Sometimes this can be costly, sometimes it may be affordable, but what it is, is convenient and by using this service you are still preparing in advance for what life throws at you during this change. You are still choosing healthier options, and being creative in what you eat.

Journaling. This lifestyle change will change your life forever. One day you will have changed so much that you may want to share your journey with others. If you decide to share, what better way to share than to go back and see how you felt each day or a few days. It is best practice to journal while you go through this journey.

Journaling can help discover what your negative triggers are, tracking your weight and measurement progress, tracking your feelings towards food, tracking your growth toward meal planning and food shopping and eating out and chosen food options, tracking your every step along the way.

Your first journal entry should note why you are doing IF and explain your goals. Sometimes people go as far as to go back to school for nutrition, or to be a trainer, life coach, and more, this journal will only assist you in tracking it all in real-time.

Your journal could be the road to success for someone or some other people who feel as though you once felt.

This can also help you when you have those hard days and want to give up, you can read back and know that I was feeling like this once before and overcame it so surely, I can again.

Journaling can only help you on this journey, it is the best practice for success.

Family Lifestyle Change. I wouldn't recommend making a drastic change, but after a few days maybe a week it's a good idea to start your family and sometimes even the company you keep around you to start eating what you eat and when you eat.

If you are the cook and shopper in your house, this will be a better use of your time. You will only have to meal plan once, shop once, and cook a few meals that will feed everyone for a couple of days.

Hopefully, this gives you more time during the week to add in exercise if you don't, or if you do maybe a second workout, or maybe give you a few hours each day to do something else you have been wanting to do, like maybe writing a book.

Brush your Teeth Earlier. Everyone should brush their teeth before bed each night. With intermittent fasting, it's better to practice brushing your teeth after your last meal. The taste of toothpaste and/or Listerine should keep you from wanting to do any further eating. This is just a mind trick, but it has been a successful helpful trick that I still use.

How to Order at Restaurants. Know the menu before you go. I repeat, know the menu before you go. Most restaurants, even fast-food restaurants, have websites on which you can view their menu options.

If you know what's on the menu before you go, you can be proactive in deciding what you will order as the best option for you.

Have a few staple times that most restaurants offer: grilled salmon, chicken breast, shrimp, and seafood, fried chicken wings with no breading or sauce, burgers wrapped in lettuce, salads, and more.

Most restaurants DO NOT serve appropriate portions of food. This is an advertising mechanism for the restaurants, it is an effective way for them to get you to continually come back and spend money with them. I mean who wants to go to a restaurant that serves those small plate options.

Most restaurants serve 2 and sometimes 3 times the portion that a person should be eating in one sitting.

To ensure you spend your money wisely but getting the food you pay for, while simultaneously ensuring that you are using good portion control, when you order at a restaurant it is good practice to go ahead and ask for a to-go plate and when your food arrives, split your food up by keeping an appropriate portion to eat now and package away from the other 2 or 3 servings for later options.

Lunch Bag Prep. Every evening after dinner, clean the kitchen and prepare for the next day. This includes preparing my lunch bag for the next day. I add the following to my lunch bag each day. 2 full meals, 3-4 snacks, and 2-3 bottles of water and sparkling water.

Although most days, I eat dinner at home, what if I didn't make it home in time to eat dinner, or what if football practice goes long, what if traffic is a mess due to an accident, what if I must work late, what if, what if, what if.

Always be prepared and you will be successful. I have had unplanned events, which have forced me to eat in the car, and sometimes dinner is a few healthy snacks because I didn't have my meal with me. Be prepared.

How to Deal with Unplanned Events. Although unplanned life events occur, sometimes 3-4 times a week, as an intermittent faster you still need to have a plan for the unplanned.

Always have that lunch box/bag with you as previously mentioned. Know a few staple food options that are your go-to food options when you are on the go and don't have your available food options.

Think before you eat always. Peer pressure is real, especially at social events, be sure to have a serious conversation with family and friends so they know you are serious and that they should not offer you items when it is not your feeding window and that your new lifestyle is not a joking matter and that you would appreciate they take it as an important part of your life.

Make good decisions and be proud of those decisions that you make. Now and then, I change my feeding windows for social events. I sometimes fast longer so that I can push my feeding window back to be able to attend social events and have dinner and drinks with family and friends.

Buy in Bulk. You may be thinking how is buying in buck related to intermittent fasting. It is vital for beginner and sometimes long-time intermittent fasters to always have food on hand to accommodate any cravings and their feeding windows.

It is best practice to buy favorite snack foods in bulk if available.

When you buy these items in bulk you can then use small ziplock and/or sandwich bags to create your serving size (according to the food label) baggies to keep in your car, purse, backpack, at school, at work, in your gym bag, in your lunch box or bag, and more.

It saves you money to buy in bulk than to buy individual items already prepackage, companies charge more for convenience, so when you buy prepackaged small cute individually packaged items it costs more than buying in bulk and doing this yourself.

This also ensures that you are only having a serving or 2 according to the food label. This also saves you from not being prepared and eating unplanned food items.

Consistent Routine. Appetite is trainable because it is driven by routine. Our bodies know and learn our routines, we are usually hungry when we expect to be hungry, not necessarily when we are physically hunger, again it could be that we are bored or need fluids.

Practice makes perfect, right? Fasting is a skill that with intermittent fasting you are trying to advance this skill.

The best practice would be at least to start with a good routine new life as you endure this lifestyle change. That means to set your alarm and wake to start most days at the same time, specifically during the week to start.

Eat your first meal and 2nd meal at the same time, you can have your snacks at whatever time during the feeding window. It is also best practice to workout at the same time of the day most days and take measurements, pictures, and weigh yourself on these same days.

Meal plan the week before you will shop and cook the meals. Then shop on the same day, and cook and prep the meals on the same day so you start the week always with good habits.

Conclusion

Intermittent fasting is very lenient as far as nutrition is concerned. By being lenient means, you are not restricted from eating anything in particular.

You can eat pretty much anything within reasonable limits once in a while. It means if you have to attend a birthday party of a friend or any other celebration, then you wouldn't have to think a million times before having a piece of cake, or any other dessert.

You can enjoy a piece without carrying the burden of guilt upon yourself. However, this liberty comes with a caveat. You must eat it within reasonable limits.

This liberty helps in keeping the temptations away. People who are tied under restrictions in eating often feel depressed and crushed.

It leads to pessimism and negativity. Remember, intermittent fasting is less about what you eat, and more about when you eat.

As long as you are following the fasting hours, your body will be able to bear the once-in-a-while indulgences. Intermittent fasting 16/8 limits the number of hours within which you can eat.

It can mean a lot for people who have a habit of snacking frequently. An intermittent fasting schedule would limit the number of meals you can take, and hence, you will have to draw your whole nutrition from 2-3 meals within the 8-10 hours eating window.

Moving on from one meal to another can get difficult if you are not having balanced meals. If you are consuming too many refined carbs, then also, you might find it difficult to move on from one meal to another without feeling the food cravings and hunger pangs.

Therefore, you must have a very balanced meal.

Intermittent Fasting 16/8

Written by Jenna Dawson

page intentionally left blank

CPSIA information can be obtained
at www.ICGtesting.com
Printed in the USA
BVHW040019040221
599227BV00009B/1094

9 781801 143103